Cambridge Elements ≡

Elements in Health Communication
edited by
Louise Cummings
The Hong Kong Polytechnic University

W0227453

CLINICAL COMMUNICATION

The Ideal of Patient Empowerment and the Reality of Patient Vulnerability and Dependence

Peter Salmon
University of Liverpool

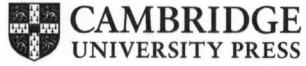

CAMBRIDGE
UNIVERSITY PRESS

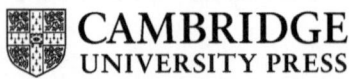

Shaftesbury Road, Cambridge CB2 8EA, United Kingdom

One Liberty Plaza, 20th Floor, New York, NY 10006, USA

477 Williamstown Road, Port Melbourne, VIC 3207, Australia

314–321, 3rd Floor, Plot 3, Splendor Forum, Jasola District Centre,
New Delhi – 110025, India

103 Penang Road, #05–06/07, Visioncrest Commercial, Singapore 238467

Cambridge University Press is part of Cambridge University Press & Assessment,
a department of the University of Cambridge.

We share the University's mission to contribute to society through the pursuit
of education, learning and research at the highest international levels of excellence.

www.cambridge.org
Information on this title: www.cambridge.org/9781009619554

DOI: 10.1017/9781009343152

First published 2025

A catalogue record for this publication is available from the British Library

ISBN 978-1-009-61955-4 Hardback
ISBN 978-1-009-34312-1 Paperback
ISSN 2754-1045 (online)
ISSN 2754-1037 (print)

Cambridge University Press & Assessment has no responsibility for the persistence
or accuracy of URLs for external or third-party internet websites referred to in this
publication and does not guarantee that any content on such websites is, or will
remain, accurate or appropriate.

Clinical Communication

The Ideal of Patient Empowerment and the Reality of Patient Vulnerability and Dependence

Elements in Health Communication

DOI: 10.1017/9781009343152
First published online: January 2025

Peter Salmon
University of Liverpool
Author for correspondence: Peter Salmon, psalmon@liv.ac.uk

Abstract: Good communication is necessary for good clinical care, but defining good communication has been surprisingly difficult and controversial. Many current ideas that identify good communication with certain communication behaviours, or 'skills', were ethically inspired to help doctors see beyond disease to the whole patient. However, promoting specific behaviours is problematic because communication is contextually dependent. In recent decades, observational research into practitioner–patient relationships has begun to provide a scientific basis for the field, identifying patients' vulnerability and practitioners' authority as defining features of fundamentally asymmetric clinical relationships. Future educators can learn from research that explores the judgements that experienced practitioners make when they manage communication dilemmas arising from this asymmetry. In future, instead of the current emphasis on teaching communication behaviours, educators could provide practitioners with knowledge about relationships to inform those judgements, while addressing the attitudes and values that motivate and guide their communication.

Keywords: clinical communication, communication skills, attachment, patient dependence, patient decision-making

ISBNs: 9781009619554 (HB), 9781009343121 (PB), 9781009343152 (OC)
ISSNs: 2754-1045 (online), 2754-1037 (print)

Contents

1 Introduction

Communication between health practitioners and patients is the vehicle for delivering clinical care. So good communication underlies good care, and research has pointed to many different pathways whereby good communication can improve outcomes – from patient satisfaction to mortality [1]. For instance, how doctors communicate influences how much patients trust them, which in turn affects patients' commitment to treatment and, ultimately, whether the treatment works or fails. Clinical communication is therefore an exciting research field and communication teaching has become a core component of pre- and post-qualification curricula in medicine, nursing and other clinical professions. However, this field remains very confusing and controversial. In particular, it has proved surprisingly hard to agree just what *is* 'good communication'.

1.1 'Good' Communication: Perspectives from Deontology, Consequentialism and Virtue Ethics

To set the scene for debates that will recur in later sections, we need to distinguish three approaches to deciding whether communication (or, indeed, any behaviour) is 'good' [2]. One is to identify specific communication behaviours as inherently good. We shall see this approach in the concept of 'communication skills' (Section 5), which denotes behaviours such as making eye contact, offering empathic statements, or summarizing what has been said as intrinsically valuable ones that practitioners should therefore be taught to use. This takes a philosophical position called ***deontology***, whereby the quality of an action is inherent in the action. From this perspective practitioners might, for example, smile and greet patients to open a consultation because they have been taught that these are the correct behaviours to start an interaction. We shall see through the following sections that deontology has been the dominant approach in clinical communication; professional, governmental or institutional guidance tells practitioners how they should communicate in different situations, published curricula tell educators which communication skills they should teach practitioners to use, and communication rating scales evaluate practitioners' performance of those skills. Even 'pocket cards' are available to tell practitioners how to communicate in specific situations[1]. In Section 4, we shall see that some very influential frameworks of guidance for clinical communication – 'shared decision-making' and 'patient-centred care' – also take an essentially deontological position in providing instructions for how to communicate,

---

[1] https://medicine.dal.ca/departments/core-units/pgme/communication-skills/communication-skills-pocket-cards.html.

procedures and materials to help practitioners follow those instructions, and assessment methods to measure how well they do so. However, we shall also see that it is very hard to create behavioural rules that cater for every situation that can arise in clinical care.

In the current era of evidence-based medicine, practitioners are expected to treat patients using methods justified by evidence of their effects. In clinical communication, too, educators and researchers therefore now often cite outcome evidence – showing, for instance, that when practitioners communicate in certain ways their patients are more satisfied or recover more quickly. This takes a ***consequentialist*** approach, whereby the consequences of a behaviour determine whether it is good. From this perspective, practitioners who smile and greet their patients might do so because they have seen evidence that it improves patient satisfaction or adherence to treatment recommendations.

A consequentialist approach to clinical communication is not straightforward, however, because any element of communication rarely has a single outcome. For instance, providing medication or treatment that patients request might enhance their satisfaction, but at the cost of iatrogenesis if the requested treatments are harmful, or of wasting scarce resources where they are pointless. This is not just a theoretical risk. Later, we will see surprising findings where doctors taught to communicate in ways that improved patients' satisfaction achieved poorer clinical outcomes for those patients [3]. Unfortunately, communication researchers have prioritized 'soft' outcomes, such as patients' satisfaction or mood, over 'hard' clinical outcomes. Indeed, the relatively small-N designs of most communication research, while powerful enough to detect large effects on soft outcomes, have insufficient power to detect the smaller effects that should be anticipated on more distal outcomes of morbidity and mortality. Even if outcome evidence from larger-scale studies were available, however, translation from such studies to practitioners' moment-to-moment communication with individual patients leaves much to the practitioners' interpretation and judgement (see Sections 5, 6). So good communication cannot simply be defined as that which achieves the best outcomes.

Just as in ordinary life, clinical communication can express values. For instance, we expect practitioners to be polite to patients, regardless of whether they have been told to be polite, and regardless of any evidence that politeness influences outcomes. Politeness indicates respect, and patients meeting rude or discourteous practitioners would feel devalued. And we expect practitioners, not only to respect their patients, but to be genuinely interested in them and motivated to discover what they need and how best to help, even in the absence of trials comparing outcomes between motivated and bored practitioners. Similarly, we expect practitioners to be knowledgeable and capable of good judgement, without waiting for evidence that knowledge and judgement improve care. Recognizing this dimension to clinical communication leads us to the third philosophical stance for identifying good communication: *virtue ethics* [4].

This approach, with origins traceable to Aristotle in the West, and Confucius in the East [5], means shifting our focus from communication behaviours and their consequences to communicators' character and to the motivations, attitudes and knowledge that underlie their judgements about how to communicate [6]; that is, communication behaviour is good where it is chosen wisely, for good reasons. From this perspective, practitioners would smile and greet patients, not because they have been taught to or because they expect better outcomes, but because they respect and value them. The critiques in this Element will return us repeatedly to the conclusion that a virtue ethics perspective is a better fit to clinical communication than is the current emphasis on deontology and consequentialism. We shall see, though, that a virtue ethics perspective does not simplify educators' or researchers' tasks. Indeed, it exposes dilemmas that an exclusive focus on behaviours and their consequences does not. For instance, how we communicate indicates who we are as people – our personality and our values. So can we change practitioners' communication without changing in some way who they are as people? Conversely, when practitioners are taught to communicate in a new way, are they no longer being 'authentic'? We return to these dilemmas later (Sections 6, 7), when we examine how the authenticity that both patients and practitioners seek in clinical relationships can be reconciled with practitioners' need to learn new ways to communicate with their patients.

1.2 What, and Who, Is This Element For?

The aim is that readers are informed and critical about this field. They need to be ready to evaluate claims they might read about communication in policy documents, research literature or educational material; and they need to be able to critique their own communication or communication that they experience or observe. So the Element is not just for academic readers. In informing practitioners and stimulating them to be critical, it can help them be more flexible and creative in finding solutions to challenges in communicating with their patients. The Element therefore takes a different stance from that of many existing textbooks on communication for doctors and other healthcare practitioners. Rather than a manual of communication skills, it is an introduction to 'clinical communication science' with the aim that clinical communication can sit alongside other clinical subjects in being founded on good science while also grounded in clinical reality [7].

The first sections therefore focus on basic principles that underlie the questions that clinical communication researchers ask or the goals that educationists choose, disentangling different influences that have shaped these principles. Reflecting the ethical dimension of clinical communication, Section 2 begins with principles that arise from ethical perspectives. Section 3 turns to principles derived from scientific models, and to the theory and research that allows us to critique these models. Section 4 critiques principles that have arisen from some communication 'technologies' that have shaped communication research and education and that have embedded in the field assumptions about how practitioners should communicate. Section 5 addresses how the technology of communication skills teaching has sought to implement those assumptions.

It is, though, of little practical use to think about principles in only general terms. Scholars applying virtue ethics to practitioners' clinical interactions draw on Aristotle's warning that the wisdom to make good judgements exists, not as theoretical or technical knowledge, but in making good judgements in practice [8,9]. Similarly, the medical anthropologist, Arthur Kleinman, argued that abstract principles remain vague generalizations with little real-world purchase unless they are tested and honed by studying what they mean in routine practice [10]. Section 6 therefore uses cancer care as a 'case study' to examine in detail what the principles identified in the preceding sections mean in clinical practice. Cancer care poignantly focuses the vulnerability and dependence that will emerge through this Element as central to the patient experience and to the psychological challenges of clinical communication. Moreover, cancer care has been an intense focus of communication research, guidance and education for more than fifty years. It therefore illustrates well the beliefs and assumptions that motivated and guided the pioneers in clinical communication research and education, and the ways in which these are challenged by more recent research. Finally, Section 7 identifies some pointers to how, responding to these challenges, the future of communication education might diverge from its past.

The field of clinical communication is vast, so this short Element is necessarily highly selective. It focuses on themes related to patients' vulnerability and dependence, thereby arguably putting what defines being a patient at its centre. And it emphasizes the practitioner–patient relationship as the vehicle for responding to patients' vulnerability and as the context within which the many functions of communication must be achieved. It is therefore a 'primer' for readers who will go on to consult literature and texts about those functions and who can read about them in light of the ideas introduced here.

Of all the health professions, doctors have historically been the main target of communication research, guidance and teaching; so most of the material cited here will be about doctors or aimed at them. Nevertheless, roles are changing, and other professions, such as nurses, physiotherapists or pharmacists, can also take clinical responsibility for patients' care. Therefore, this Element, although informed mainly by literature concerning doctor–patient relationships, is potentially relevant more broadly to professionals consulted by patients seeking clinical expertise in response to feelings of vulnerability associated with physical disease. For clarity, the text will refer explicitly to doctors only when citing evidence or guidance that specifically concerns them. Elsewhere, the generic term 'practitioner' will indicate the potentially wider relevance of the material or ideas in play. Ultimately, it is for readers to make their own judgements about the extent to which ideas in this Element apply to their own context. The central thesis of the Element is that understanding 'clinical communication science' can equip readers to make good judgements, whether about communication in clinical practice, communication teaching, or communication research.

2 Ethical Context: What *Should* Clinical Communication Be Like?

Current priorities in clinical communication research and education can be understood as reactions to the authority that doctors have exerted over their patients for millennia. From the earliest recorded accounts of illnesses and their remedies, patients have sought help from people with authority to recommend or administer treatments [11]. In the West, Egyptian medicine linked physical wellness to spiritual health, so physical illness could be caused by wrongdoing that offended spirits or gods. Authority was thereby built into healers' role: the authority, not just of specialist knowledge and experience, but of association with supernatural power. Similarly, prominent Eastern systems of medicine were linked closely to beliefs about metaphysical influences on the body, so treatments came with the authority of those who interpreted the supernatural world [12].

In the face of healers with access to hidden forces, patients could not expect to understand or influence what was done for them; their role was to accept what they were told. Once developing empiricism gave rise to more physically based theories of illness, doctors became distinct from priests and magic [11]. But they retained the authority associated with their specialist knowledge; clinical relationships continued to be shaped by the expectation that patients accepted what doctors told them. Reflecting evolving expectations of an increasingly industrial and consumerist society, the twentieth century finally saw powerful challenges to the culture that became known as 'medical paternalism' [13,14]. First, legal changes began to constrain doctors' authority and establish patient rights.

Secondly, from bioethics and social science, and from within medicine itself, new ideas arose to put patients at the centre of clinical care, and to increase their authority over what doctors do to them and for them.

2.1 Patient Self-Determination: Legal Frameworks of Informed Consent

The beginning of legal constraint on doctors' authority was marked by a judgement in a New York court in 1914 [15]. The case did not change law, but changed how existing law was interpreted in a new age of developing medical technology and changing societal expectations about individual rights. It arose because a patient sued a surgeon whose intervention had gone beyond what the patient had previously agreed to. Having accepted examination under anaesthesia the patient awoke to discover that the surgeon had identified and removed a tumour. Side effects of surgery led to circulatory problems that later necessitated amputation of some of the patient's fingers. The eventual ruling stated that *'every ... adult ... has a right to determine what shall be done with his [sic] own body; and a surgeon who performs an operation without his [sic] patient's consent commits a battery'*. In other words, it equated treatment without consent with being physically attacked. Since this landmark judgement, the principle of 'informed consent' has evolved, albeit at different speeds in different countries. In general, the criterion for 'sufficient information' evolved from the information that a 'reasonable practitioner' would give to what a 'reasonable patient' would expect. In the UK in 2015, a landmark legal case moved the criterion further; for a patient to be adequately informed of the risks of treatment, the practitioner must tell the patient, not only what a 'reasonable patient' would consider important but what that *specific patient* would think important [16]. Practitioners need, therefore, to be able to detect and respect the values and concerns of each patient, an injunction to which we will return repeatedly in this Element.

The trend towards respecting patients' *'right to determine what shall be done with his own body'*, in the words of the 1914 judgement is, in practice, highly constrained by culture and politics. For instance, in seeking to reject treatment that prolongs life, or to request intervention to end life, there are intense contests when patients or families draw on evolving cultural views of individuals' rights in the face of legal constraints and religious or political opposition [17]. Similarly, the United States illustrates how decades of extension of women's rights over doctors in relation to contraception and abortion can rapidly be reversed when political power shifts. Aesthetic surgery, where patients seek surgical solutions for psychological reasons, remains highly contentious, with laws sometimes enacted to constrain patients' access to certain procedures [18].

Contest over individuals' rights in relation to doctors arises also when states seek to mandate interventions. For instance, across Europe different legal frameworks around mandating or encouraging vaccinations against contagious diseases in children [19] and (in light of the COVID-19 pandemic) adults [20] reflect contrasting cultural and political views of health as an individual or collective responsibility [21,22]. Clearly, the *'right to determine what shall be done with [one's] own body'* cannot be understood simply according to a linear progression from medical paternalism to patient emancipation. Self-determination in practice has proved more nuanced than envisaged in the idealized statement from the New York court.

2.2 Patient Self-Determination: The Bioethics of Autonomy

The cultural trends that led to legal assertion of patients' rights have been expressed in academic and professional perspectives on clinical relationships and we shall see that these, too, illustrate the practical complexity around respecting patients' rights as autonomous individuals. In Section 3 we will see also how, within medicine itself, new ideas were arising that centred clinical care more on patients' needs than on their doctors' traditional priorities (Section 3). And in Section 4, we will see how social scientists took up the cause of patient empowerment, thereby aligning patients with other groups marginalized by powerful interests. First, though, we address how bioethicists' ideas about 'patient autonomy' evolved as a moral foundation for those developments; and we shall see that the initial simplicity of an idealized view has evolved into a more nuanced picture.

Beauchamp and Childress' famous statement of the principles of ethical clinical practice [23] enshrined respect for patient autonomy as one of doctors' canonical ethical obligations. Autonomy was equated with self-determination; patients need the information that equips them to decide for themselves about their treatment and care, and they should make such decisions freely, without coercion. By being enabled to make treatment decisions, patients were defended from the dangers associated with medical paternalism – that decisions would reflect doctors' preferences or assumptions instead of individual patients' values and needs. With hindsight, however, it became clear that asserting patients' right to self-determination brought problems. For instance, where they seek interventions that would be pointless or harmful, or that might squander scarce healthcare resources, acquiescence adheres to the principle of autonomy but contravenes Beauchamp and Childress' other fundamental principles: beneficence (provide what is in patients' interests), maleficence (do not harm patients) and equity (treat all patients according to their need). Taken to the extreme, an over-riding emphasis on patients' self-determination could replace paternalism by consumerism, whereby doctors are reduced to offering a cafeteria of services from which patient-customers can select [24]. While the lens of consumerism might help illuminate limited areas of clinical practice such as aesthetic surgery, in which requests for clinical intervention can reflect social and cultural factors as well as personal needs [25,26], we will be concerned here with patients whose need for care is defined by feared or confirmed physical disease.

Equating patient autonomy with self-determination presents a further difficulty; it is rare that patients or their families are psychologically equipped to make good decisions. First, the worry or distress associated with being mortally ill, or with the fear of being so, are inimical to the rational and objective judgement that clinical decisions need. Second, it is implausible that patients could routinely be brought to the level of understanding and judgement necessary for complex clinical decisions, that practitioners take many years to reach. In Section 4 we will examine the concept of 'shared decision-making' (SDM), designed to help patients be self-determined in a context in which they lack technical knowledge and expertise or find it hard to reason objectively. However, more recent developments in bioethics suggest that aiming for self-determination as the way to respect patients' autonomy is mistaken.

Concern with self-determination expresses a normative element of Western culture: the valuing of individual decision-making and responsibility. By contrast, in some other cultures, important decisions for individuals are made in groups of which they are a part, particularly the family [27]. Even in the West, the value attached to self-determination is not so robust that it can survive the threat of mortal illness, as a Canadian study showed strikingly more than three decades ago. Degner and Sloan [28] asked two samples of people to rate the degree to which they would want to make decisions about treatment for cancer or have their doctors make decisions for them. The sample of healthy people, asked to imagine needing treatment, predominantly sought to be in control of decisions. By contrast, the sample of people recently diagnosed with cancer mostly wanted the doctor to be in control. The study's message is that being mortally ill changes how we value personal control. It makes us look to practitioners to take care of us, rather than to our own sense of self-determination.

There is another reason to be cautious about taking too literally the value attached to individual responsibility and self-determination in the West. It probably tells us more about self-presentation than about people's wish to be self-determined. That is, it is culturally valued in the West to appear – and feel – in control of one's own life. Therefore, when patients are asked in questionnaires or interviews whether they want to be informed and to make decisions about their treatment for themselves, they typically say 'yes' [29,30]. But this probably reflects what a *New England Journal of Medicine* editorial called an 'information-as-power ethos', rather than a true desire for information and choice [31]. In Section 6 we shall see that patients (or, where patients are children, their parents) who present themselves as wanting to be fully informed and to make decisions for themselves go on to describe needing their doctors to constrain information and take responsibility for decisions. Therefore we should be wary when self-report questionnaire studies appear to confirm patients' desire for information and choice [32]. Some questionnaires simply tell us about language [33]. For example, when patients endorse questionnaire items to indicate that they want 'enough time' to make decisions [30] the simplest explanation is that, in English, it is impossible to say that one does not want enough of something! Practitioners are often advised to give patients 'the information they want to have', but asking patients what they want to know is clearly not straightforward. Responses to such a question are fundamentally uninformed; patients cannot make informed decisions about what information they want until they know what that information is [31].

Western individuals' health-related decisions that, at first sight, seem to be expressions of self-determination based on individual preferences, such as the choice to be vaccinated for COVID-19, can on closer scrutiny be seen to have a strong relational element; individuals' choices reflect social relationships and obligations and broader cultural influences [34]. Reflecting the need for an understanding of autonomy that does not simply recycle cultural norms around self-determination, Western bioethics literature has seen growing interest in ideas of 'relational autonomy' [35–38]. Originating in feminist critiques that equating autonomy with self-determination depicted individuals as unrealistic-ally self-sufficient and isolated from a social network, relational approaches emphasize the social and cultural context within which people make choices. From a relational perspective, therefore, individuals' autonomy can arise, not from making decisions for themselves, but from being able to rely on other people who respect, value and understand them and on whom they can depend to make decisions that are right for each individual.

A relational perspective has big implications for how practitioners might respect patients' autonomy. Most strikingly, asking patients or their families to make choices could even *reduce* autonomy. In a report pointedly entitled 'Autonomy gone awry', Orfali and Gordon [39] compared parents' experiences of neonatal care between France and the United States. In France, satisfaction with care, and a sense of personal autonomy, arose out of a strong doctor–patient relationship based on a traditional emphasis on medical authority and responsibility. By contrast, in the United States, with care characterized by greater emphasis on parental decision-making, parents were less satisfied, felt less resilient after the loss of a baby, and felt poorer rapport with doctors. Compared with an approach to autonomy that equates it with self-determined decisions, a relational view invites many other ways to respect patients' autonomy. For instance, we shall see (Section 6) that, when doctors give reasons for their treatment decisions, patients can better 'own' those decisions [40,41]. Moreover, a relational view takes us beyond decision-making for other ways to enhance autonomy. It points to mundane aspects of social interaction that communicate respect and dignity instead of disrespect and arrogance, such as being polite and well-prepared, acknowledging patients as equals, taking seriously what patients know or apologizing when late [42–44]. From a relational perspective, patients' autonomy does not, of course, just require patients to trust their practitioners to understand and look after their interests; it depends on practitioners genuinely being trustworthy in understanding and respecting each patient's interests and in having the expertise to address them. As Pellegrino explained, '*the vulnerability and dependence of the sick person forces him [sic] to trust not just in his rights but in the kind of person the physician is*' [45].

Whereas relational autonomy marks a change of direction for Western bioethics, it converges with long-established perspectives in less individualistic cultures [46]. For instance, Nakata et al. [47] showed how the concept of 'motenashi', embedded in Japanese society, could inform bioethics of critical care, but their paper is relevant more broadly. According to motenashi, people who are respected should not be burdened with the expectation or obligation to make decisions to secure what they need. As Nakata et al. explain, '*The respected person does not have to make any decisions because decision-making is always accompanied with risks and responsibilities.*' Rather, the obligation is on others to know what they need and to provide it. As a cultural practice, motenashi obliges hosts to discover and to respect what will satisfy and please their guests. As a bioethical principle, it obliges practitioners to understand and respect what matters to their patients. It therefore shows clearly why a relational approach to autonomy does not presage a return to paternalism, whereby decisions reflect what suits practitioners or what practitioners think best.

2.3 Conclusion

Redressing the imbalance of power between patients and practitioners from a legal perspective has proved more complex than a simple, linear process of patients taking ever more of practitioners' power for themselves. Similarly, autonomy in bioethics is not a 'zero sum' whereby practitioners must simply cede authority for patients to gain it; the concept of relational autonomy is more nuanced than the earlier equation of autonomy with self-determination. Recognizing this complexity does complicate this Element's task. Equated with self-determination, patient autonomy is relatively straightforward to deliver; practitioners give patients the information they need to make decisions about their care and allow them to make those decisions freely; educators can therefore promote patient autonomy by teaching practitioners the behaviours necessary to inform patients and share decision-making with them. Understood in this way, respect for autonomy would belong in deontology ethics; practitioners achieve ethical practice when they perform certain behaviours. By contrast, relational autonomy is not reducible to behavioural rules. Instead, it points to a virtue ethics perspective because it concerns the qualities that practitioners must have; not only clinical expertise and wise judgement but the motivation and ability to understand and respect what matters to each patient.

3 Psychological Theory: What *Is* Clinical Communication Like?

3.1 The 'Psychotherapeutic Model' of Clinical Communication

While the historical paternalism of medical care was being challenged in society and in bioethics, there were challenges from within medicine too. In 1977, a US psychiatrist, George Engel, advocated a revolution in medical thinking and practice [48]. Engel criticized medicine for being 'doctor-centred' or 'disease-centred', marginalizing patients' emotional and social needs and their preferences and concerns. He blamed two fundamental principles of medical thinking. 'Reductionism' was the belief that everything that mattered in clinical care was biological and ultimately explicable at the molecular level. 'Dualism' was the assumption that the patient's body and mind were separate and that doctors needed only to concern themselves with the body. Opposing these principles, he advocated a 'biopsychosocial model' of clinical practice, which recognized that both the causes and effects of illness often lie outside biology, being found instead in interactions between patients' biology, psychological processes and social context. It followed, he argued, that doctors needed to be concerned, not just with their patients' physical symptoms, but with the social and psychological context of those symptoms. They needed to understand, for instance, how patients' emotional state, beliefs or social circumstances might be causing or exacerbating illness, and they needed to address the psychological and social consequences of the illness. Engel's attempt to change the culture of medical care by centring it on the whole patient instead of the biological disease helped set the scene for subsequent development of practices to implement 'patient-centred care', to involve patients in decision-making, and to teach practitioners to be more holistic in their communication, to which we turn in Sections 4 and 5. Here, we examine how views about the nature of the clinical relationship evolved following Engel's paper.

Key pioneers of clinical communication research and teaching were, like Engel, psychiatrists or with training in psychology or social science. They therefore brought a professional concern with patients' psychosocial worlds which, when applied to care of patients with physical illness, offered to help implement the biopsychosocial model. From their perspective, the clinical relationship is an emotional connection. It develops over time as practitioner and patient get to know each other, being built through emotional talk just like relationships in psychiatry or counselling; the practitioner shows concern with the patient's emotional feelings, the patient discloses them, and the practitioner in turn responds empathically [49]. On this reasoning, the strength of the relationship, and the degree to which it comforts distressed patients, depends on this emotional talk rather than on instrumental talk about the illness and treatments. This view of clinical relationships became very influential and continues to shape assumptions and practices in clinical communication education and research. Indeed, it is so influential that it is widely seen as axiomatic, and rarely identified in clinical communication literature as a contestable theory. However, we need to examine the validity of extending this model from the psychiatric or counselling clinic to the very different context of clinical relationships in physical illness.

The extent to which this 'psychotherapeutic' model of clinical relationships shaped researchers' and educators' expectations of practitioners' communication is illustrated by a consensus statement in 2010 by European clinical communication experts [50]. In explaining why oncologists should receive communication training, it states that they often disregard the emotional and social dimensions of their patients' illness, and that their preference for focusing discussion on medical information can be a way to avoid such talk. Common research themes in clinical communication, and the language with which findings are reported, also illustrate how the psychotherapeutic model has become 'taken for granted'. For instance, many papers have reported on the level of empathy that doctors show their patients, lamenting their failure to show enough. In one influential paper, Levinson et al. [51] reported on the number of cues to personal issues or emotional feelings that were present in patients' talk when they consulted surgeons or primary care doctors. By describing these cues as '*opportunities*' for the doctor to '*demonstrate understanding and empathy*' and thereby '*deepen the therapeutic alliance*', they reveal how they think that those doctors should respond: in English, an 'opportunity' is not a neutral word, but indicates the expectation that it should be grasped. The key finding was that doctors responded empathically to 38 per cent of cues in surgical consultations and 21 per cent in primary care. The authors' language again goes beyond scientific observation to indicate that the doctors had fallen short. For instance, *'frequently [doctors] missed opportunities to adequately acknowledge patients' feelings'*. Words like 'miss', 'opportunity' and 'adequately' all add rhetorical power to the argument that doctors failed. But the paper does not specify to what extent they failed; it does not state whether, for instance, doctors should respond empathically to 100 per cent of empathic opportunities, 50 per cent or some other proportion. The reason is that there is no evidence to indicate what a desirable percentage should be. Their conclusion also disregards whether the doctors responded by addressing the clinical problem that elicited the cues [52], for example, by providing relevant information [53]. Similarly, many researchers have shown that communication training can increase practitioners' demonstrations of empathy [54], but without specifying a target level. Simply assuming that more is always better seems implausible, and closer to a slogan than a scientifically grounded prescription. In the limiting case, it might absurdly predict that the strongest clinical relationship would be achieved by exclusively emotional talk that disregards clinical care.

The apparent face validity of the psychotherapeutic model when applied to clinical relationships in physical healthcare therefore belies some conceptual difficulties. Scrutinizing the model further reveals several reasons why it does not clearly fit healthcare for physical illness. First, the suggestion that clinical relationships in this setting need an explicitly emotional connection between practitioner and patient is questionable. After all, practitioners need to be dispassionate and objective with their patients, not emotionally involved [55], and need effective clinical relationships even with patients whom they dislike. The performative language often used in educational or research literature seems to acknowledge this problem in its frequent reference to 'displaying' empathy, rather than 'being' empathic, thereby degrading the concept of an emotional connection to something enacted rather than felt. Moreover, the overwhelming emphasis on empathy risks encouraging practitioners merely to respond empathically to patients' emotional cues without first identifying what gave rise to them and what practical responses might be needed [56].

A further limitation of the psychotherapeutic model is its oversimplification of relationships [57]. First, emotional and instrumental communication are not as distinct as the model assumes. Emotional needs can be communicated and addressed by factual talk, and vice versa [58,59]. For example, patients can secure general practitioners' (GPs') clinical engagement with their symptoms by emphasizing how worried or upset they feel [60], and patients with advanced cancer mentioned the death of a loved one after oncologists failed to respond to previous clues to their need to talk about their own impending death [61]. Second, in everyday life, relationships are multidimensional and often asymmetric; the different parties to a relationship can feel different levels of connection. Literature and drama poignantly exploit the divergence that can arise between the sense of relationship felt by each party (love unrequited, for instance), and it is obvious that a strong relationship can exist in the absence of explicitly emotional talk. By its 'one-size-fits-all' approach, the psychotherapeutic model simplifies relationships in another way. It has little to say about how they vary between different contexts; for example, how they differ between clinical settings, between surgeons and nurses, or amongst individual patients and individual practitioners.

Finally, and crucially, the psychotherapeutic model disregards the defining feature of clinical relationships in physical healthcare: the inherent asymmetry of vulnerability, knowledge and authority when patients are – or fear being – physically ill [62]. Patients are typically suffering or frightened, and consult practitioners who they believe have the knowledge and authority to help them. In this context, the more plausible starting point for understanding clinical relationships is that patients' main priority is not their emotional feelings, but the health problem provoking those feelings.

3.2 Attachment Theory and the Clinical Relationship

Instead of importing a psychiatric model of clinical relationships into physical medicine, we need a way to understand these relationships that is better suited to their very different context. Recently several writers have drawn on attachment theory, which has asymmetry of vulnerability and authority at its centre [49,63–65]. The theory emerged from studies of children with their parents [66,67] and centres on a simple observation that, when a child feels vulnerable, its overwhelming priority is to be close to a familiar caregiver – usually the parent. The parent is its 'attachment figure', or 'secure base', that helps the child feel safe and cared for. The child has an emotional bond with the parent, called an attachment. Crucially, attachment figures are not substitutable; if one is not available, someone else with whom the child has not formed an attachment would not suffice. Attachment theory is not just a theory of dependence; the security provided by an attachment figure who is available and attentive is the basis for the child feeling confident to explore and become independent. For instance, a young child taken to a nursery by a parent might run off and explore, but will periodically look back at, or return to, the parent, confirming that the world is still safe to explore further. The convergence with the earlier discussion of ethical theory is clear; autonomy when one is vulnerable depends on being able to trust in others' authoritative and attentive care.

Although originating in studies of childhood, attachment theory has been applied also to close relationships in adulthood, particularly in the context of vulnerability as a powerful trigger for attachment processes. However, attachment relationships for adults differ in many ways from those seen in children [68]. With adulthood comes the ability of symbolic representations of the attachment figure to substitute for proximity; for example, the promise of an impending meeting with the attachment figure, or just knowing that he or she is available [69]. In some situations, adults can also need appropriate distance and separation to find a sense of safety [70]. Most obviously, parents generally give way to other attachment figures – in particular, romantic partners. However, adults can compartmentalize needs for different kinds of support; different people might offer a 'secure base' but in relation to different sources of vulnerability. Moreover, whereas being comforted is usually the main indicator of safety for a child, adults seek more evidence of the authority of a potential attachment figure to ameliorate threats. Therefore, given the vulnerability inherent in physical illness, or the threat of it, patients can see a practitioner as having properties of an attachment figure in providing a 'secure base' in the context of the threat of illness [65]. Several implications for clinical relationships follow from this reasoning, and they diverge greatly from those of the psychotherapeutic model.

First, it is primarily practitioners' authoritative and expert biomedical care, not their emotional engagement, that allows patients to see them as a 'secure base'. Therefore, a practitioner who focused too much on patients' worry would probably be harder for patients to see as a 'secure base' than one who focused authoritatively and expertly on the symptom or disease causing the worry. Therefore patients can prefer doctors to respond to their emotional cues with practical clinical information rather than with emotional talk [53]. Of course, there will be situations where patients need practitioners who are explicitly empathic, and who spend time exploring their feelings and concerns, particularly in primary care where GPs often have to disentangle confusing presentations of physical and emotional symptoms. But, as the *starting point* for thinking about how practitioners comfort patients, attachment theory points in a very different direction. Consistent with an attachment perspective, we shall see in Section 6 that practitioner behaviours that allow patients to see them as attachment figures do not resemble the psychosocial exchanges advocated in the 2010 consensus statement described previously [50]; instead patients identify behaviours indicating expertise, authority and commitment, and patients or family who feel in emotional turmoil can sometimes need practitioners who provide a secure base by being calm and rational instead of engaging with their distress [71] (see Box 1).

Healthtalk (https://healthtalk.org) curates an on-line library of patient accounts of illness and treatment. Navigate to this patient's interviews: https://healthtalk.org/interviewees/interview-09-7/ Three interviews illustrate how a practitioner's ability to provide a 'secure base' is influenced by their communication: (i) In the interview entitled 'He felt safe in the hands of a surgeon who spoke frankly', the patient is comforted in the face of bad news when a surgeon shows genuine authority and commitment; (ii) In 'A sympathetic visit from his surgeon … ', the patient describes feeling intensely comforted ('like therapy') because the surgeon came to sit with him and talk after an operation that failed to reverse his colostomy. (iii) By contrast, in 'Describes being wrongly told he had only a short time to live', we see him feeling abandoned by a doctor who showed no commitment to take care of him when giving bad news.

From an attachment perspective, therefore, patients' sense of emotional connection to practitioners does not need to arise over time from explicitly emotional talk. Rather, it arises out of patients' vulnerability and associated attachment needs and their ability to see the doctor as a secure base. The multidimensionality of relationships (which the psychotherapeutic model does not easily accommodate) therefore becomes understandable; patients' sense of emotional connection is not based on observable emotional engagement, or on reciprocal emotional feelings in the practitioner. Indeed, attachment theory helps us understand how a strong emotional connection for patients can arise from practitioners' conscientious clinical care, whereas clinical communication educators and researchers have generally portrayed clinical care and emotional engagement as distinct [72]. Recognizing this exposes a danger for practitioners who, misled by not feeling that they have an emotional relationship with a patient, do not appreciate the intensity of connection that the patient can feel to them. They risk shattering patients' ability to construct them as a secure base where they do not display conscientious and authoritative care, for example, by failing to honour promises to a patient, forgetting a patient's name, not being well-informed about a patient or appearing uninterested in the patient or family [62,73].

A 'secure base' does not mean a practitioner who makes unrealistic promises to cure a patient or remove pain. Instead, it signifies the practitioner's commitment to be with the patient through the challenges of illness and not to abandon the patient. Therefore, what makes a practitioner a 'secure base' depends on the context. For instance, a study of palliative care patients being cared for at home identified aspects of care that helped patients and their families feel they had a 'secure base' when cure was impossible [74]: knowing that practitioners were available, seeing the same ones rather than unfamiliar faces, and feeling that the practitioners respected the patients and their families by listening and taking their concerns seriously. Even during the COVID-19 pandemic, when practitioners often had to provide support remotely, by telephone, it was possible for patients or family members to feel that a practitioner was 'with' them when the practitioner addressed clinical care conscientiously and authoritatively [75,76].

An attachment perspective also helps understand heterogeneity amongst patients in the way that clinical communication supports clinical relationships. In the acute crisis of a frightening illness or diagnosis, most patients' concern will be with their practitioners' ability to take the role of authoritative and conscientious attachment figures. Later, to learn effective and confident self-management as a long-term condition proceeds, patients will need practitioners who, while still being trusted to be authoritative and available, also respect and value patients' own developing perspective and authority. Moreover, patients' readiness to form trusting relationships will be influenced by their childhood experience of attachment [68]. In general, a child experiencing attentive and consistent care and affection will be better prepared as an adult to enter close, trusting relationships than one without that experience. More specifically, according to attachment theory childhood experiences can independently shape adults' assumptions about other people and about themselves when in close relationships. These sets of assumptions are sometimes called 'mental models' [77,78], and each can be positive or negative to different extents. The model of 'others' is what the adult expects of other people: being trustworthy, caring and considerate where the model is positive, or untrustworthy, uncaring and rejecting where negative. The model of 'self' is what people feel about themselves. The positive end of this dimension denotes feeling deserving of care and affection; at the negative end people feel unworthy, even unlovable. Putting these two mental models, or dimensions, together, yields a classification of 4 attachment styles [79] (Box 2). Using questionnaires to categorize attachment style, around half the general population fall into the 'secure' category, defined by positive models of both self and other, the other half being distributed across the remaining styles [80]. Differing communication needs between patients can reflect these attachment styles (Box 2). Patients whose experiences have left them distrustful of other people (negative model of 'other') will need sensitive prompting to disclose symptoms or concerns. Patients who have learned to feel unloved, or unworthy of care and affection (negative model of

Box 2 Adult attachment styles and clinical relationships

Adults' mental models of self and others vary from negative to positive, defining four attachment styles. Names here are according to Ciechanowski [79], replacing traditional (and pejorative) terms in brackets. For each style, text illustrates implications for patients' relationships with practitioners (see 64, 81, 84).

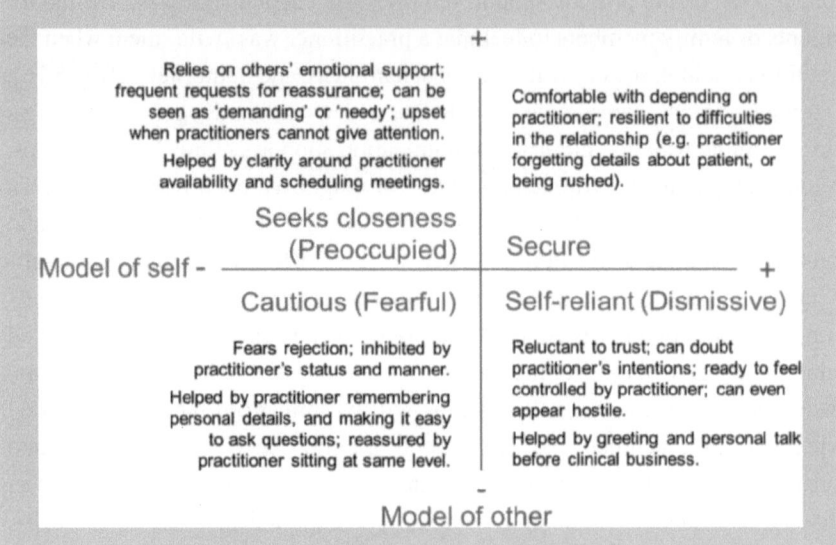

'self'), will need more reassurance than do others that their symptoms and concerns are important to practitioners and will be taken seriously. Patients hardest to reach will be those in the 'cautious' quadrant, where both models are negative, and some might need expert psychological help [64,81–84]. Evidence that patients with one of the 'insecure' attachment styles reported a poorer relationship with their doctors than did 'secure' patients [85] is a warning about the additional help that these patients need to form trusting relationships.

Attachment theory also alerts us to heterogeneity between practitioners. Because their capacity to be a 'secure base' depends on their power and authority in the face of patients' vulnerability, attachment theory is most obviously relevant when patients see physicians or surgeons in the context of a physical health crisis. We should not expect clinical relationships with other professionals, or in other situations, to arise in the same way. Indeed, there is evidence from interviews with nurses and oncologists that they support patients emotionally in contrasting ways; the oncologists relied on clinical expertise and authority to comfort patients and families, while nurses engaged at a more explicitly emotional level [86]. Of course, heterogeneity amongst practitioners arises, not just from different professional roles, but from their own attachment styles and the experiences that shaped them. For instance, there are reports that medical students with 'secure' attachment style achieved higher scores in assessments of clinical communication [87] than did other students, and were more likely to choose careers in primary care than in hospital specialities, perhaps indicating greater comfort with a specialty that emphasizes long-term relationships with patients [88]. There is evidence, too, that doctors' attachment style predicts aspects of their responses to patients' presentation [89–91], and even patients' presentation itself [92]. For example, a doctor who has learned to be wary of emotional closeness might seek distance from patients who show dependence. However, the demands of professionalism mean that patients should not be at the mercy of practitioners' different attachment styles. Instead, practitioners have the responsibility to appreciate how their attachment style influences their clinical relationships and, as part of learning their professional role, to become able to transcend this style when necessary. Of course, practitioners vary in ways that are not captured by formal assessments of attachment style, and patients can value idiosyncratic aspects of individual doctors' presentation [73]. After all, to offer a secure base a practitioner needs to be a committed individual, not just acting a role.

Attachment theory is, like any other psychological theory, an imperfect lens through which to see what might otherwise be obscure, and it is important not to use it inappropriately. While it might help understand some differences between practitioners in their response to patients, or how they cope with the challenges of clinical care [93], it cannot explain *why* they care [49]. For instance, to claim that, because practitioners enjoy relationships with patients and can feel upset when patients suffer or die, they have attachments to their patients [94] is implausible. For a patient, the practitioner is non-substitutable as an attachment figure, but practitioners must be ready to move on to the next patient without the burden of grief-like responses when one patient suffers or dies. As a paediatric oncologist explained in a qualitative study, '*We are sad at the time [of giving bad news of treatment resistance] and then we have to move on because we have other patients waiting for us*' [95]. Extending attachment theory to explain practitioners' caring risks recycling the implausible assumption of the psychotherapeutic model: that clinical relationships are a symmetrical emotional connection between practitioner and patient.

Attachment theory is, of course, not the only theoretical lens available to view clinical relationships. From psychoanalytic theory, the concepts of 'transference' and 'counter-transference' have been used to describe how patients and practitioners, respectively, can transfer feelings or attitudes from previous relationships onto a current, clinical one. Similarly, 'projective identification' describes how one party to the relationship can take on emotional feelings, such as helplessness and hopelessness, emanating from the other. Kelly et al. [96] illustrated how these concepts can help to understand doctors' clinical decisions in end of life care. A practically oriented application of psychoanalytic theory arose in the 1950s. Named after the psychoanalyst who first developed them for GPs, 'Balint groups' were small groups of doctors, facilitated by a leader but drawing on peer-supervision to help analyse and understand challenging clinical relationships [97]. Balint argued that the clinical relationship could even have a therapeutic function [98]. These groups continue, albeit outside the mainstream of clinical communication practice and research [99], and without clear evidence about outcomes [100]. Arguably, the language and theory of attachment will be more accessible than psychoanalytic theory to practitioners who are not psychological specialists.

3.3 Conclusion

This section, on the *science* of clinical relationships, has converged with the conclusion of the previous one, about the *ethics* of relationships. Each began with an idealized view that excluded the inherent asymmetry of expertise and vulnerability that defines clinical relationships. And each has concluded with a way of understanding clinical relationships that is built on that asymmetry, and that sees practitioners' authority as the basis of the relationship. Both science and ethics therefore point to a serious dilemma: patients remain inherently vulnerable, regardless of the quality of practitioners' communication. It is well known that vulnerable children or adults can be abused or exploited by powerful individuals whom they trust. Similarly, patients' need to trust a 'secure base' leaves them open to abuse and exploitation. They can even become impassioned supporters of ostensibly authoritative practitioners whose clinical peers denounce them as fraudulent and exploitative [101]. In the extreme case, practitioners whom patients trust as strong attachment figures can even be murderous. Patients described one GP in the UK as 'going out of his way' to look after them, but he murdered hundreds [102]. Because vulnerability and dependence are inherent in clinical relationships, ensuring that patients are protected from care that is paternalistic, or even exploitative or abusive, cannot be delegated to patients themselves by a deontological emphasis on practitioners' performance of communication behaviours such as providing information and offering patients choices about treatment decisions; it remains the practitioners' responsibility. This Section therefore points, once again, to the need for communication teachers and researchers to engage with practitioners' character, including their knowledge, values and motives [6].

4 Technologies of Patient Empowerment and Patient-Centredness

Here, we turn to the work of social scientists and others who sought to guide practitioners and educators to implement the biopsychosocial approach to care that Engel advocated in 1977 [48]. They developed sets of principles and practices that resemble 'technologies' in that they include specified ways of communicating, techniques and materials to promote those, and measurement procedures to assess how well practitioners' communication conforms to the specifications. These technologies draw on scientific ideas and methods, particularly in evaluation studies, but arguably they cannot be said to be truly 'evidence-based' because very little inductive evidence about the nature of clinical communication was available to inform their development. Instead, they arose as essentially morally motivated efforts to humanize medical practice. This section addresses two influential and overlapping sets of technologies concerned with enhancing patients' empowerment and involvement in their healthcare and centring care on the patient rather than the disease. The science and ethics of clinical communication have been changing, as we saw in previous sections; so we must scrutinize these technologies in light of the knowledge and theory that has arisen since they became established as defining features of the landscape of clinical communication research and education.

4.1 Patient Empowerment

While recognition of the persisting paternalism of medical care motivated bioethicists' interest in patient autonomy, it also drew social scientists' attention to patients' role in healthcare. The broader context was the growing social and political concern with empowering marginalized groups in society. Here we examine related technologies that arose out of concern with patients' empowerment in healthcare and with ensuring their involvement in healthcare decisions.

4.1.1 Measuring Empowerment: Patient Enablement and Activation

Social science is notoriously a field in which multiple, competing theoretical frameworks arise and fall out of fashion rapidly. Unsurprisingly, therefore, many overlapping theories and models have arisen under the broad heading of patient 'empowerment' or 'engagement'. The result is a confused field, containing a profusion of imprecisely defined concepts and associated procedures for their implementation and assessment, albeit linked by a belief that patient empowerment means being equipped and motivated to take responsibility for one's health and to make self-determined decisions about healthcare [103–106]. Two of these concepts have had particular influence, reflecting the development of self-report questionnaires that made them measurable: 'patient enablement' and 'patient activation'. 'Enablement' usually refers to what practitioners do to enhance patients' capacity to shape their care, although it sometimes refers to that capacity itself. By contrast, 'patient activation' usually signifies a property of patients: a readiness to take control of their health and healthcare that comprises not just capacity to shape care but also motivation to do so. The questionnaires developed to measure each concept have stimulated quantitative research on their outcomes for patients and on the factors that can enhance empowerment by increasing enablement or activation.

Outcome research focusing particularly on patients with long-term conditions finds that those with higher scores on measures of activation or enablement are, in general, better-adjusted to their illness, cope better with symptoms, make less demand on emergency care, have better biomarkers of health and illness, and do better clinically [107–113]. On examining items of the most widely used questionnaires, however, it becomes clear that such associations need to be interpreted cautiously, particularly where, as in most studies, they are based on cross-sectional rather than prospective designs. For instance, items of the questionnaire widely used to measure enablement ask about the extent to which respondents feel confident about keeping themselves healthy and coping with illness [114]. Clearly, higher scores will be more likely where people's experience is of illness that is less serious and more easily treatable or manageable by the patient. The same difficulty applies to several items of the main questionnaire used to measure patient activation, endorsement of which indicates that patients feel that their health is mainly under their own control (see, for example [115], Box 3).

While evidence of an *association* of patient outcomes with activation or enablement cannot prove *causation*, experimental studies potentially provide stronger causal evidence by testing the effects of interventions designed to increase patients' capacity and motivation to take responsibility for their own healthcare. The most significant clinically have been for people with long-term conditions, reflecting these patients' need to manage their conditions autonomously over time without day-to-day medical supervision [116]. That such interventions improve clinical outcomes is shown by many reports, exemplified by those of Kate Lorig in the United States in diabetes and other conditions [117]. The influential 'Chronic Care Model' [118], originating in the United States but now guiding service provision for people with long-term conditions

Box 3 Patient activation

These links help to explore how the concept is implemented in practice.

https://www.ncbi.nlm.nih.gov/pmc/articles/PMC1361049/ [115] This paper describes the development of the 'Patient Activation Measure' (PAM), explaining that a measurement instrument allows healthcare providers to be held to account for their efforts to increase activation. It describes what an ideally 'activated' patient can do, including self-management, collaborating with practitioners and even selecting health-care providers by researching and weighing up evidence of their quality.

https://www.insigniahealth.com/ This company markets a widely adopted measure of activation. Cost-saving for organizations that adopt patient activation is the first of several promised benefits. Note the language of the labels for the four categories into which patients' PAM scores categorize them. The version of the questionnaire in common use is not directly available on this website, but can be found in recent articles (e.g. https://www.ncbi.nlm.nih.gov/pmc/articles/PMC7735884/). The confidence about managing one's illness that many of the items measure tells us about the attitudes of patients who endorse them; but might endorsing these items also indicate something about the nature of their health problems?

in many other countries [119], therefore explicitly includes the enhancement of patients' self-management as an essential element in improving their care, along with the service reorganizations needed to support this. However, although self-management interventions can increase activation or enablement, it is not clear whether patients' attitudes to self-management are the crucial contribution to improved clinical outcomes. The programmes have many other potentially beneficial components, such as stress management and exercise promotion [120]. Even where statistical modelling shows that changes in patient attitudes can account for improved outcomes, findings should be interpreted cautiously. For instance, a recent report of exercise training for diabetic patients showed that increases in activation were related to improvements on emotional and physical variables, but the variance explained was very small (3–8 per cent) and might even result from an influence of the outcomes on activation rather than vice versa [121].

These interventions typically include encouragement of patients' adherence to goals that professionals have set for them; for instance, Lorig's diabetes programme includes instruction to monitor blood glucose or think positively

[120]. It is hard to reconcile directing patients to expert-specified goals with a view of patient empowerment as self-determination. By contrast, from a relational perspective there would be no contradiction in patients being empowered by being helped to comply with professionals' expectations of them, provided those expectations truly reflect each patient's own interests. Moreover, there is evidence that patients feel more empowered when care is better, i.e. when doctors are more empathic, give longer consultations and take a more holistic approach [122]. That is, if healthcare services look after patients better, patients feel better able to look after themselves. This echoes our conclusion after examining ethical theories of autonomy in Section 2; patients' autonomy depends on being well cared for by people who respect their needs and values. Recall, also, attachment theory in Section 3: being able to depend on a trusting relationship with a secure base is the foundation for developing the capacity and confidence to be independent in managing a health condition.

There is danger, however, in the enthusiasm with which the language of empowerment has been adopted by healthcare organizations and politicians apparently unaware of, or unconcerned with, its relational context. Selling programmes of patient activation is now a business, driven in large part by a commercial organization (Box 3). The key measure of patient activation is copyrighted, and services pay to use it. Patient empowerment is being advocated, not just to improve patient outcomes, but as a way to save healthcare organizations money [123]. If those two outcomes are aligned, there is no conflict between them. But the danger lies in the risk that those organizations or the governments that fund them seek, under the guise of 'empowerment', to devolve responsibility for meeting patients' needs to patients who are ill-equipped for that responsibility [38,124,125]. The danger is patent in absurd claims by both politicians and academics that, for example, patient empowerment has allowed patients to 'control their medical destiny' [126,127]. This politicization of empowerment is paralleled in the morally loaded language of what should be a scientifically based field. For instance, patients with the lowest scores on the Patient Activation Measure are widely categorized as '*disengaged and overwhelmed*' or '*becoming aware but still struggling*'; those with the highest scores earn the more complementary label '*maintaining behaviours and pushing further*' (e.g. [128], Box 3). These labels, arguably, go beyond description to convey moral value: higher scores identify people who merit approval for having taken responsibility. Similarly, in many academic papers, enablement or activation are regarded as 'clinical outcomes' in their own right, as if they are inherently valuable rather than being merely putative mediators of real patient benefit. It seems that moral and scientific reasoning are apt to become entwined in this field.

4.1.2 Shared Decision-Making

Also drawing on ethical ideas around autonomy, the technology of 'shared decision-making' (SDM) has provided more explicit guidance about how practitioners could contribute to patients' empowerment by involving them in decisions about their own care. Although the principle of sharing decisions with patients had been advocated for decades, the technology of SDM began to take shape in the 1990s [129,130]. Its aims were to respect patients' autonomy (understood from the ethical perspective of self-determination), and to ensure that decisions about treatment are consistent with each patient's needs and values. SDM recognized that, for example, some patients might give a higher priority to certain side effects of a treatment than other patients – or doctors – would or, conversely, that some patients might be ready to tolerate treatments that others would consider too onerous. The aims of SDM could be delivered, it was argued, by following some general principles. First, patients and practitioners should share information – the patients about their symptoms, needs and priorities, doctors about treatments and their risks and benefits. Second, they should both participate in decision-making. Third, they should agree a final decision. Arguing that these principles were vague and open to variable interpretations in practice (for instance, around what exactly 'participate' means, or 'sharing' information), Elwyn et al. proposed more practical recommendations [131,132]. First the patient should know that a choice exists, and that therefore a decision is needed. Second, he or she should know what the options are and what their effects are. Third, the patient should deliberate – that is, should think about the options and weigh them up. Turning to the practitioner, Elwyn therefore described several kinds of talk that are needed: explanation that a choice exists; description of the options; and support to deliberate and agree a decision [133].

SDM has been widely endorsed by healthcare organizations. Nevertheless, the objective features of shared decision-making remain elusive in routine practice [134,135]. Its failure to penetrate practice has prompted re-examination of the recommendations for SDM specifically, and of the concept of patient involvement more generally, identifying several difficulties [135–141]. First, to follow the guidelines can be laborious for practitioners, who might simply have insufficient time, and who can have multiple decisions to make in a single consultation [142]. It can be burdensome for patients, too, who often do not want to deliberate about treatment options or feel unqualified to. While valuing being recognized by practitioners and healthcare institutions as individuals used to making decisions for themselves, the main decision patients make in a clinical context can be about trusting their clinical team rather than choosing treatment. Similarly, they can look to their practitioners' personal judgement and experience as information resources more valuable than the objective information emphasized in SDM [125]. In this way, patients can feel involved, but having 'reinterpreted' involvement to mean following expert guidance [143]. Moreover, although Elwyn et al. specified their recommendations to achieve SDM in some detail, they remain imprecise. For instance, it remains unclear exactly what 'deliberation' means; it might even include thinking irrationally or inaccurately.

Accounts of SDM also lack recognition that it does not remove the reality that clinical relationships are asymmetric; practitioners inevitably usually have more knowledge and experience than they can share with patients, and patients' vulnerability can leave them emotionally ill-equipped to make difficult decisions, to the extent of needing to trust experts to do so. Therefore, as we shall see in Section 6, patients can gain a sense of partnership with doctors from receiving information, even when they take no part in decisions (Box 4). Even where there are options, it is still the practitioner who constrains choice by deciding which ones to offer. In many situations, moreover, no real choice exists – there is only one clinically justified option – so SDM procedures would have little value. Moreover, the emphasis on agreeing the final decision does not address situations where patients need to be persuaded; for instance, where they seek treatment that will be ineffective or harmful, or where they reject potentially life-saving treatment out of concern about relatively minor side effects.

Finally, SDM shares the limitations of models of decision-making that were influenced by the assumption that people make decisions rationally and that there is therefore usually an objectively 'good' decision to be deduced [141]. In reality, people routinely make important life decisions by using 'heuristics' which 'short-

---

BOX 4 INFORMATION SUPPORTS PARTNERSHIP

This set of interview extracts on Healthtalk illustrates patients' varied expectations and experiences of decision-making (https://healthtalk.org/experiences/shared-decision-making/what-shared-decision-making/).

The sixth patient describes having a strong sense of 'partnership' with his cardiologist. But this is based, not on having shared decision-making with her, but on the cardiologist taking responsibility for decisions while explaining each one to the patient. Other patients explain the importance of doctors knowing what matters to the patient and of respecting patients' own expertise, particularly in managing long-term conditions where expertise arises from the patients' experience of self-management.

cut' decision-making [137]. In particular, they often make choices by following the recommendations of someone whose expertise they trust, or they decide emotionally according to how different options 'feel'. Decisions that depend on these 'gut feelings' and other heuristics can be efficient and accurate, perhaps partly because the decision-maker avoids information overload [144]. Nevertheless, people's habitual use of heuristic decision-making presents problems for SDM. First, patients are liable to be unprepared to deliberate about options in a novel, rational way [125]. Second, identifying what is an objectively 'good' decision becomes elusive because non-rational, heuristically based decisions are apt to be idiosyncratic and contextualized [137].

The development of rating scales to measure the extent to which SDM is present in consultations fuelled research which identified another difficulty with the concept. High inter-rater reliability can be achieved between observers trained to use the same instrument [145]. However, scores from different instruments are sometimes unrelated [146], and, when patients and practitioners rate their consultations for SDM, their scores do not reliably correlate with observers' ratings, or with each other's [145]. It seems that SDM can mean different things to different people [147] (Box 5). Given these difficulties with the concept, it is unsurprising that reviews of patient

Box 5 OBJECTIVE AND SUBJECTIVE SDM DIVERGE

Saba et al. [147] (paper available at https://www.annfammed.org/content/4/1/54.short) categorized primary care consultations in a US clinic according to whether SDM was (i) present objectively in the doctor–patient dialogue and (ii) present in their subjective experience. The table shows that these two ways of classifying consultations did not correlate. Text shows some of the reasons for divergence.

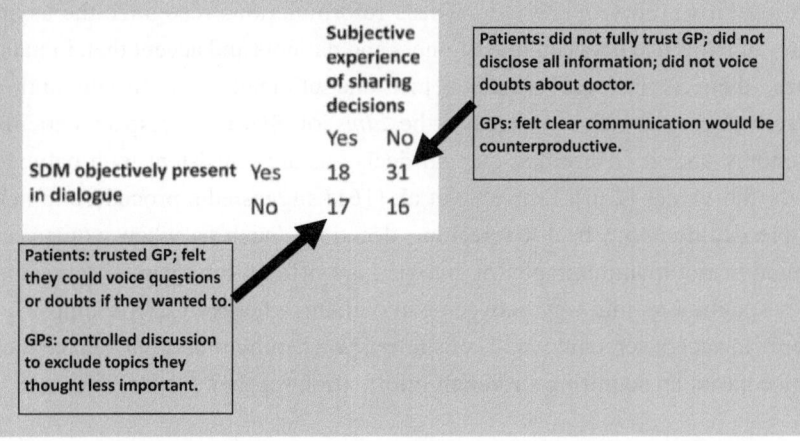

outcomes when practitioners have been trained to follow SDM guidance have not, in general, provided strong evidence of tangible benefits for patients [148–152].

While SDM has not yet appreciably changed the patterns of dialogue in routine consultations, a very tangible expression of SDM is the burgeoning availability of 'decision aids' [153]. These are instruments – on paper or on-line – designed to involve patients in care decisions by providing information about treatment options in ways that patients can understand and make use of, and by structuring patients' deliberation about the available choices. They differ greatly in format and complexity (Box 6). Some use pictograms to depict statistical concepts liable to confuse patients, for example, the difference between relative and absolute risk reduction when taking a statin drug to reduce the risk of a serious cardiovascular event. Others rely on verbal, rather than pictorial presentations. Patients who use them are better informed, have more accurate understanding of risk, feel less conflicted about their eventual decision and take a more active part in decisions [154,155]. Although it is not clear that, in general, decision aids change the decision, their use in older people might help avoid invasive life-sustaining procedures in favour of comfort care [156]. Nevertheless, like SDM dialogue in consultations, decision aids remain rare in routine practice. One practical difficulty is that, in the effort to encompass more and more of the information potentially relevant to a decision, they become longer, more complex and less easily readable, putting them beyond the reach of many patients – thereby repeating the trend seen in patient consent forms [157,158]. That some healthcare organizations or professional bodies mandate or encourage the use of decision aids to protect practitioners from accusations that they did not adequately inform patients about a procedure [159,160] points to the danger that we saw with patient activation; a technology inspired by the need to empower patients can be co-opted to serve practitioners' or institutions' interests.

In the face of these practical and conceptual problems with SDM, there have been attempts to reformulate the concept to better fit the reality of clinical relationships [136,137,139,161]. These reformulations recognize the asymmetry of expertise between practitioners and patients and accept that, in many cases, there is no real choice – just one clinically appropriate option. Nevertheless, they try to achieve the *aims* of SDM: to respect patients' autonomy and to ensure that clinical decisions are consistent with patients' needs and values [136]. Entwistle et al. [161] suggested a procedure to help people decide about health screening decisions, such as when women are offered breast mammography or smokers are offered lung cancer screening. They sought a middle way between paternalism, whereby experts simply tell people to accept screening, and consumerism whereby individuals make their choice based on acquiring sufficient information for themselves. The starting

---

Box 6 PATIENT DECISION AIDS

Developers of decision aids (DAs) must confront the tension between making them easier to use (shorter, simpler language, fewer statistics) and accurately conveying the necessary information.

At low levels of complexity, DAs simply portray risks and benefits of treatment in ways more accessible than verbal statements of probability. For instance, this brief DA (https://assets.publishing.service.gov.uk/government/uploads/system/uploads/attachment_data/file/976877/CovidStats_07-04-21-final.pdf) used pictograms to show benefits and risks of vaccination against COVID-19 for people of different ages. This DA (https://statindecisionaid.mayoclinic.org) uses similar pictograms to explain the risks and benefits of a statin drug.

During this webinar (minutes 27–38) https://www.youtube.com/watch?v=agjce7TEDJc the developer explains a DA for people offered lung cancer screening. It aims to be comprehensive, but in trying to encompass all relevant information it has become longer and more complex.

This site https://decisionaid.ohri.ca/Azsumm.php?ID=1851 links to DAs that take different communication approaches, some going beyond simple pictorial depiction of risk probabilities. One (on genetic testing for Alzheimer's disease) tries to help undecided users by using 'vignettes' of patients making the decision.

---

point for their approach is a relationship with a trusted practitioner, such as a GP, who provides a recommendation to accept a specific screening offer and explains which experts have recommended it – for example, a professional body or government-appointed scientists. The practitioner then describes why those experts made the recommendation, and why they can be trusted, before explaining how anyone who wants more information can access it. Entwistle et al.'s approach recognizes that most people want to trust experts about such a decision and that, for these people, the responsibility for ensuring that the decision to be screened is the right one must rest with those experts and cannot be devolved to the patient. It also recognizes that some people will want to be more informed.

A second proposal addressed major treatment decisions such as in cancer care [137]. Again, it emphasizes that good decisions require a clinical relationship with a trusted practitioner, who should evaluate the patient's ability and motivation to make what the practitioner would regard as a 'reasonable' decision for that patient. For example, if life-saving intervention is available with minimal risk, then the reasonable decision would normally be to accept it. If the patient is a Jehovah's Witness, however, and the intervention is a blood transfusion, the reasonable decision might be to reject it because this religion eschews transfusion. That is, the reasonableness of a decision must be judged from the patient's perspective, not the practitioner's. Practitioners should therefore assess and engage with patients' decision-making by exposing and, where necessary, challenging the propositions that guide their heuristic reasoning. They should then take the responsibility to lead decision-making, from gentle prompts through to persuasion, to the extent that patients are unable or unwilling to reach 'reasonable' decisions.

Both these approaches clearly rely on practitioners' sensitive judgement. They cannot be implemented simply by specifying behavioural rules for them to follow. Similarly, we saw that previous formulations of SDM also defied attempts to specify objectively agreed and measurable procedures. Instead, the reformulations emphasize the essential values of SDM – respecting patients' autonomy and ensuring that decisions serve patients' own priorities and values [162]. This, in turn, points to the qualities that practitioners need to develop if they are to be ready to detect and respect patients' priorities and values, including humility, curiosity and flexibility; as Piertese et al. observed, '*how can a doctor . . . explore "patient preferences" without being curious about that specific person and his/her life*' [163].

4.2 Patient-Centred Care

There have been calls to centre care on patients rather than their diseases since the beginnings of recorded medicine. However, systematic use of the term 'patient-centred care' or, more recently, 'person-centred care' [13], dates from the middle of the last century; Balint, a psychoanalyst, advocated 'patient-centred care' in urging GPs to concern themselves with the 'whole patient' [97,98] (Section 3). Current popularity of the term owes much to the work of a Canadian group of primary care researchers in the 1980s and 1990s, and to their advocacy of a 'Patient-Centred Clinical Method' [164–166]. Essentially, this guides practitioners to explore and be concerned with patients' experience of illness, and to collaborate with patients in creating a shared understanding of the illness. In inviting patients' own perspectives into the consultation, practitioners can learn from their patients and can arrive at options for care that reflect each patient's needs and values. In its emphasis on bringing patients' emotional experience and psycho-social world into the consultation, this guidance clearly follows the lead of Engel's earlier description of the 'biopsychosocial model' [48] (Section 3), and overlaps with the aims and practices of SDM. However, over recent years, both empirical and theoretical difficulties with the concept have become clear. In linking the clinical relationship to explicitly psychosocial talk, patient-centred care has less to say about the role of practitioners' expertise, authority and conscientious *clinical* care in sustaining clinical relationships. Moreover, continued refinement and reinterpretation has resulted in many different definitions of patient-centredness [13,167]. For instance, one influential UK healthcare 'think tank' defined it as care that is coordinated, tailored to the individual, underpinned by dignity, compassion and respect, and that enables a fulfilling life for the patient [168]. Essentially, this is a prescription for good quality care, and the term 'patient-centred' is in practice now widely used to mean 'good' care.

Empirically, although training practitioners to communicate in ways that characterize patient-centred care can change their communication, there have not been clear benefits for patients' clinical outcomes [169]. Indeed, one evaluation of training became famous in the field as a warning that communication that looks patient-centred might not always be in patients' best interests [3]. GPs and specialist nurses were trained in patient-centred communication, focusing specifically on care of patients with diabetes. Patients seen by trained practitioners felt more satisfied with practitioners' communication and treatment than did those seen by an untrained control group. Despite this evidence that training made consultations more patient-centred, two clinical markers (blood triglycerides and body mass index) were poorer in patients seen by trained practitioners, as was patients' knowledge about diabetes. These findings point to the danger that emphasizing the importance of a clinical relationship based on engaging explicitly with patients' emotional experience might constrain doctors' clinical care [170,171]. Moreover, there is a risk that learners reject the concept of patient-centredness where it is taught as behavioural skills without provision for them to understand the concept and to relate it to real experiences of care [172].

Once again, we see that a technology with moral aims cannot readily be sustained at the level of behavioural rules that practitioners can be taught to follow, because those rules turn out not to be inherently and consistently in patients' best interests. However, the literature and guidance that has grown around the concept of patient-centred care is important in helping practitioners to define their role more holistically than a focus on diseases decontextualized from patients' lives. That is, the value of this technology lies most clearly in the domain of values. Being truly patient-centred means having the attitudes and beliefs that define patient-centeredness: respecting and valuing patients as unique individuals. As Duggan et al. suggested, being genuinely patient-centred is *'just the right thing to do'* [2].

4.3 Conclusion

Each of the technologies in this section is a morally grounded attempt to deliver aspects of the biopsychosocial model: to ensure that practitioners respect patients as autonomous individuals with needs that extend beyond the biology of their disease to encompass its psychosocial context. Each technology offers practical solutions at the level of behaviours that practitioners can adopt: they can use specific consultation strategies to involve patients or to elicit and respond to their psychosocial needs, and they can use questionnaires to audit patients' empowerment. However, each technology does not clearly work at this deontological level; practitioners who are taught to use those consultation strategies do not always help their patients by doing so, and the questionnaires do not always detect what matters to patients. Instead, our analysis points again in the direction of virtue ethics: that involving patients and meeting their psychosocial needs depends on practitioners who respect their patients as autonomous individuals and who understand and respect their needs.

5 The Technology of Communication Skills

Like those in Section 4, this technology also seeks to implement ideas promoted in the biopsychosocial model [48] by guiding and teaching practitioners to address patients holistically; it thereby seeks to promoting the humanity, as well as effectiveness, of healthcare [173]. Its aims clearly overlap with patient empowerment and patient-centred care, and it includes techniques designed to help implement those technologies.

The term 'communication skills' emerged in academic literature around the middle of the last century, attracting interest from psychologists over subsequent decades. Psychologists' affinity for the concept reflects the reductionist epistemology that characterizes experimental psychology, resembling that of natural and biological sciences whereby complex topics are rendered amenable to study by first being broken down into smaller elements. Therefore, psychology divides the human psyche into discrete domains for study, such as cognition, skills and personality. Then those domains are divided further; for instance, personality can be divided into discrete traits, like extraversion or neuroticism, that can be studied independently. The assumption is that a complete picture can be rebuilt by amalgamating findings from discrete domains. The 1960s and 1970s saw this approach applied to understanding social interaction in the belief that this complex area could be reduced to individual behaviours, or skills, that could be defined objectively. These were called social skills or, given the central role of communication in social interaction, communication skills [174,175]. The concept of clinical communication skills is therefore inherently reductionist in conceptualizing communication and relationships as built from component skills [176]. An attraction of this approach was the implication that, once skills were identified, they could be taught to help improve communication and social interaction.

The 1980s saw rapid growth in reports of teaching communication skills to diverse social groups including medical and dental students and qualified doctors. Communication skills training (CST) gradually became an integral and, in some countries, obligatory component of pre- and post-qualification medical training [177–179]. CST has become particularly embedded in cancer care, reflecting pioneering work by social scientists, psychiatrists and psychologically minded practitioners who advocated teaching communication skills to practitioners as the key to good communication, and therefore good clinical care [180–182]. There are probably several reasons for the success with which CST has become established in clinical curricula [178]. First, in prioritizing communication behaviours to promote clinical relationships, it addressed the growing expectations that practitioners be 'patient-centred'. More controversially, CST perhaps benefitted from a social and political climate that emphasized the accountability of clinical professions, with patients increasingly positioned as consumers [178]. Indeed, some proponents of CST have been stridently critical of practitioners for their poor communication skills, and communication skills teaching and research have offered a route whereby social scientists, psychiatrists, general practitioners and others could shape clinical education and clinical practice very broadly.

In line with the psychiatric or psychological background of many pioneers of CST, curricula have emphasized skills for exploring patients' emotional feelings and for responding empathically to their expressions of emotional distress, as well as skills for effective information exchange and sharing decisions [183–187]. There are many published curricula that list skills to be taught (several including many tens of skills) although some refer to communication 'tasks' or 'competencies' instead of skills. These range widely from relatively narrow concepts such as 'eye contact' or 'ask open questions', to more diffuse aspects of clinical relationships such as 'attentive listening', 'relate to patient respectfully' or 'build an empathetic relationship'. Two opposed trends can be seen in the proliferation of these curricula. While some skills are assumed to be generalizable across professions or clinical situations [185], a parallel trend is for progressively narrower specifications of skills for specific groups, particularly oncologists [183], or situations, such as serious illness [188], breaking bad news[189] or recruitment to clinical trials [190]. The former trend assumes that the core elements of communication do not vary significantly across clinical roles or scenarios. This is hard to reconcile with our discussion of attachment theory in Section 3;

a surgeon who offers to remove a patient's cancer at first meeting, a nurse who listens to a patient's detailed worries and questions, and a GP whom a patient sees every few weeks about a long-term problem, probably all sustain their relationships with patients in different ways. By contrast, the opposing trend, towards proliferation of training of ever-greater specificity, risks becoming impracticable [191,192].

5.1 Assessing Communication and Communication Skills

Curricula often include some classroom teaching, but the emphasis is on supervised role-play and expert and peer feedback, often with actors playing the part of patients. To assess outcomes of CST the usual method is for observers to score learners' display of taught skills with real patients or actors playing patients. Many clinical communication researchers use the same approach to study communication skills in routine consultations. Although several observational coding schemes are available, they share a similar, reductionist approach in breaking down streams of communication into elements that can be quantified. The pioneering scheme was Bales' 'Interaction Process Analysis' [193,194] reported in 1950 and applied in clinical and other settings. To apply his method, an observer identified segments of speech or non-verbal behaviour that could be allocated to one of twelve broad categories; six concerned task-oriented communication (such as seeking suggestions or giving opinions) and six assessed social-emotional communication (such as showing 'solidarity' or 'antagonism'). Crucially, the observer's task was interpretive: that is, to impute the meaning, or function, of each segment of dialogue in the context of the whole interaction and of the observer's knowledge of that type of interaction. Subsequent clinical communication coding schemes have mostly followed only one of these two defining features of Bales' system. Reflecting the emphasis on overt emotional engagement with patients that we have already seen in communication literature, they continue to distinguish clinical, or instrumental, communication from communication that is emotional in content and overtly oriented to the relationship (e.g. [195-199]). The second feature of Bales' scheme, interpretive coding, has been rare in subsequent coding schemes. Instead, most have been designed to be as objective as possible in distinguishing different elements of communication according to what can be directly observed; that is, according to their form rather than imputed function. Nevertheless, accounts of these coding schemes then typically conflate form and function by equating emotional talk with emotional function and regarding communication that is task-oriented as having little relational value [197]. The pursuit of objectivity in measurement perhaps reflects the continued attraction of the natural and biological sciences as models for communication research. Sometimes this lure is explicit; for instance, when the radiological term 'thin-slice' is used to refer to coding of brief segments of clinical dialogue [200].

5.2 Critiquing the Concept of Communication Skills

Beginning in the 1980s, when the view of communication as made up of objective and teachable skills was taking shape, writers have questioned the validity of an educational model based on reducing communication to objectively definable elements that can be taught by communication experts [7,33,176,191,201–206]. First, communication behaviours do not, in practice, have universal meaning that can be objectively defined. For instance, the same behaviour from a practitioner can be perceived as caring or uncaring by different people or in different situations [207]. Behaviour that objectively provides only instrumental support can be experienced emotionally [58,59] and, when patients talk about symptoms or treatment, they can mean many different things depending on the relational and clinical context [208,209]. The reason is that communication is inherently subjective and contextual; what a listener hears depends, not only on what the speaker has said, but on the subjective and social context, including the interaction to that point. This problem is typically hidden in plain sight by communication curricula or coding schemes; when behaviours, such as eye contact, are listed as skills to be taught or counted they are usually qualified by words like 'appropriate', thereby implicitly acknowledging their contextual dependence [33]. But gauging the 'appropriate' moment to make or avert eye contact, to speak or be silent or to touch a patient depends on sensing the 'atmosphere' of a consultation that defies reduction to individual elements and which the practitioner is simultaneously both sensing and shaping [176,210]. Moreover, many listed 'skills' are global aspects of relationships, such as 'empathy' or 'partnership', which are clearly not objectively definable behaviours. Other aspects of communication that defy an attempt at behavioural description are simply absent from curricula or coding schemes. For instance, we shall see in Section 6 that qualitative researchers who examine clinical communication in cancer care induct-ively have identified potentially valuable communication practices that are missing from published lists of skills. One influential framework for communication teaching and assessment does therefore emphasize the attainment of communication goals (SEGUE: Set the stage, Elicit information, Give information, Understand the patient's perspective, and End the encounter), leaving learners to decide how to achieve each [211]. This approach arguably shifts reductionism to another level; the function of the whole consultation is understood as the aggregate of these predefined component functions. However, goals in consultation can be complex and idiosyn-cratic, changing rapidly from moment to moment [212,213].

An important consequence follows from recognizing the invalidity of the assumption of objectivity in communication. Communication skills research, and the evaluation of CST, rely heavily on quantitative research designs; correlational studies link the quantity of specific types of communication to patient outcomes, while randomized trials test effects of training on practitioners' performance of skills. However, because the same behaviour in different contexts can have different meanings, designs that aggregate measurements of communication behaviours across consultations or patients can be of only limited help to practitioners. For instance, many studies quantify practitioners' empathic behaviour, correlating it with patient outcomes like satisfaction, or showing that CST increases empathy. But the value of empathic behaviour depends, not on its quantity, but on its nature and timing, so counts of empathy tell us little. Similarly, a single well-chosen utterance can change the mood of a whole consultation – the 'lucky punch' that Langewitz described [214]. For several decades, there have been warnings that, because of this inherent variability and subjectivity in communication, the findings that quantitative outcome research can deliver are inevitably limited to bland generalizations [33,215]. Consistent with these warnings, reviews of the outcomes of CST have consistently shown little clear evidence that patients benefit – even when practitioners' behaviour changes in line with what was taught [216–220].

An even more fundamental problem with the concept of communication as made up of skills is rarely acknowledged in academic literature, although poignantly illustrated by a BBC news report of the launch of communication training for doctors in the UK NHS.[2] In drafting the headline '*Doctors to get lessons on being nice*', the journalist pointed with humour to the tension between learning caring behaviours and being authentically caring. That is, while patients and practitioners value authenticity [221] (Section 6), learning to display caring or empathic behaviours is not the same as being authentically caring or empathic. Educationists and ethicists identify the conundrum; predetermining objectives for students' learning means that, when students deliver these, their performance cannot be regarded as self-determined, but self-determination is necessary to view behaviour as authentic [8,222]. Some clinical communication research continues to disregard this challenge (e.g. [223]), and communication skills literature has not yet offered a theoretical framework within which learning skills can be reconciled with authenticity (Box 7).

Despite these difficulties with the concept of communication skills, it still shapes many educators' goals. The educationist, Eisner, echoed Winston Churchill's statement that '*we make our buildings and then our buildings*

---

2 http://news.bbc.co.uk/1/hi/health/1952712.stm.

_{BOX 7 COMMUNICATION SKILLS TO ENHANCE PATIENTS' TRUST?}

Based on patients' evaluations of video-recorded vignettes of acted consultations that were identical except for small variations in what the 'oncologist' told the 'patient', the authors of this study [223] (https://www.sciencedirect.com/science/article/pii/S0923753419365093) concluded that:

> *'Oncologists can strengthen their patients' trust by adapting their communication behaviour. This finding should encourage oncologists to express their competence, honesty, and caring behaviour and should be addressed in oncologist communication skill training. Enhancing patients' trust requires only a few seconds.'*

Their suggestion raises an ethical dilemma. Teaching behaviours that enhance patients' trust by indicating practitioners' expertise and caring locates the quality of practitioners' communication in those behaviours. In contrast to this deontological approach, a virtue ethics approach would emphasize that doctors need to *be* expert and caring.

make us' when he warned that *'we make our curriculum and then our curriculum makes us'* [224]. That is, behaviours defined as 'skills' come to define good communication. After all, the word 'skill' itself implies something to be valued intrinsically. Similarly, the availability of communication coding schemes, particularly where there is a technologically sophisticated interface that makes it easy and attractive to use,[3] shapes and constrains the questions that researchers ask. Therefore, in evaluations of CST, learners' performance of taught skills is typically presented as sufficient evidence of successful training. Papers that become widely cited as demonstrating the value of CST show increases in the quantity of skills displayed in real or simulated consultations without any evidence from patients' perspective [225,226]; increased performance of skills is sufficient for communication to be described as 'improved'. In this way, researchers and educators, rather than practitioners or patients, define what is valued in clinical communication, even to the extent of berating practitioners' routine communication and asserting their continued need to be trained to use expert-defined communication skills [227].

This problem matters because, as we shall see (Section 6), patients can value aspects of communication other than the skills that communication experts value and measure [53,228,229]. Therefore, when patients evaluate consultations, their

---

[3] For an illustration of one very widely used system, see: www.youtube.com/watch?v=Iv8wbiwYYv8.

evaluations do not correlate appreciably with those of communication experts based on practitioners' performance of skills [230,231]. There has long been suspicion that the focus on expert-defined skills might ill-serve patients' needs. Algedahl et al. [232] studied video-recordings of consultations with hospital doctors in Norway, concluding that the doctors were 'courteous but not curious'. In other words, they had learned to perform the skills of courteous, polite interaction with patients, but were not authentically interested in them and in what made them, and their healthcare needs, unique. The authors warned that more CST would not solve this problem. We saw in Section 4 that training for diabetes practitioners that focused on patient-centredness skills left patients more satisfied with consultations but with poorer biomarkers [3]. Similarly, the only statistically significant outcome of one CST programme for practitioners caring for end-of-life patients was that their patients were more depressed than those cared for by untrained practitioners [233]. While unexpected findings like these might be 'Type 1 errors', or 'false positives', they are warnings that CST might even sometimes have deleterious effects by focusing practitioners on their own performance of skills at the expense of their patients' needs.

In shaping what educators and researchers value in clinical communication, the communication skills model also risks narrowing their gaze. By attributing failures in communication to lack of skills, it promotes a 'deficit' model; that practitioners lack certain skills which they need to be taught. But this stance can blind researchers and educators to other reasons for apparent communication failures. After all, most practitioners probably already have learned much about communication and relationships before they start clinical training, and might have other reasons for not drawing on what they know. For instance, they can *decide* that certain 'skills' are clinically inappropriate or unnecessary in some situations [234], or do not fit their feelings about the patient or their own mood [235] or their view of their professional role [236]. Patients can trigger emotional reactions in practitioners that stop them using skills they have or that even lead to collusion with patients to avoid certain issues [237–240]. Many common complaints about practitioners' communication potentially indicate attitudes that signify lack of respect, or arrogance [43,44]. Perhaps attributing such behaviours to 'lack of 'skills' helps avoid the more brutal implication that some practitioners do not respect their patients and feel superior to them.

5.3 Breaking Bad News

Breaking bad news repays detailed attention because it has been a major focus of teaching and guidance over decades and illustrates poignantly the main elements of the critique in this Section. Reflecting its importance, and many practitioners' nervousness about the task, several protocols have been published to guide practitioners. The most influential is known by the acronym SPIKES [241], signifying six broad sequential tasks (Setting up, Perception, Invitation, Knowledge, Emotions with Empathy, and Strategy or Summary). It provides detailed instructions for how to achieve each task, and scripted illustrations of the necessary communication skills, including making empathic statements. However, several critics have argued that such protocols are unrealistic [228,242–245]. They define bad news as objective information and assume that consultations containing it can therefore be predicted in advance and standardized or controlled by the practitioner. However, the subjectivity of bad news means that practitioners cannot always anticipate it. For instance, some patients with persistent and troubling symptoms find being told that tests or investigations found *no* serious abnormality distressing – the 'bad news that nothing is wrong' [246]. Moreover, bad news is rarely a single piece of information in the way that the protocols assume. It often arises as one more event in a sequence: doctors tell the patient that they are concerned; they explain that further tests are needed; then one of those tests shows a need for more tests; then perhaps there is a diagnosis; then a proposal for treatment; but then perhaps the treatment cannot start for a few days or weeks; then there are blood tests or a scan that show an initial effect of treatment; then there are further results, with implications for changing treatment and so on. Each point in the trajectory of information can reveal what feels like bad news to the patient; so bad news can be a continuous and subjective process rather than a single objective event. Therefore, Eggly [243] argued that patients' interpretation of information as bad news should be seen, not as an objective fact *instigating* consultation, but as a subjective inference *emerging from* it, and from the relationship within which the consultation occurs. Moreover, Langewitz [242] warned that bad news can confront both practitioners and patients with '*existential questions that push both persons to the limits of what they can bear*'. If consultations about bad news are not so amenable to practitioners' control as protocols suppose, it is unrealistic to assume that they can be programmed to unfold in a consistent way.

Protocols for breaking bad news also illustrate the danger of scripting practitioners' emotional support. Illustrations in SPIKES of empathic statements include explicitly referring to the news as 'bad', and citing the practitioner's own emotions, for example in being 'sorry' to have to give the news, or finding 'it very difficult for me also' [241]. We shall see in Section 6 that these are strategies that some cancer doctors have told researchers that they would never use [247,248]. Indeed, Langewitz [242] suggested that a list of what *not* to say might be more helpful than attempts to specify what *should* be said. Moreover, the focus on emotional talk and empathic statements could be at the expense of clinical information that, as we saw in Section 3, patients might find more comforting [244]. Box 8 points to a consultation acted according to guidance contained in protocols such as SPIKES, prompting the reader to question whether such a scripted approach is necessarily what patients need. In contrast, Box 9 points to an account of a patient who gained an immediate sense of having a 'secure base' from the four words with which her surgeon introduced the news of a cancer diagnosis.

Despite these difficulties, once protocols such as SPIKES become widely adopted, the skills and practices that they advocate become 'taken-for-granted', illustrating how expert-defined communication skills become the 'gold standard' for communication. Therefore, there remains very little evidence as to whether patients benefit when practitioners follow such protocols because, as with communication skills training generally, researchers have been content to show that, unsurprisingly, training practitioners to follow a protocol increases their adherence to the protocol [249,250]. Frameworks such as SPIKES might be helpful to new or uncertain practitioners. However, their 'gold standard' status is hard to justify.

5.4 Methodological Shortcomings of Quantitative Communication Skills Research

It seems that training in communication skills in general, and breaking bad news specifically, continues on a path that it is not well grounded empirically or theoretically, a phenomenon that would be recognized as a serious failure of evidence-based medicine in other clinical specialties. The reason may lie in the

---

BOX 8 BREAKING BAD NEWS

'An excellent encounter': https://www.youtube.com/watch?v=_uOS7hfKkVI This video (played by actors) illustrates how to follow recommendations, such as those in the SPIKES protocol [241], when breaking bad news. The 'doctor' greets the patient politely; she displays empathy, even sympathy with the patient's emotion, and expresses her own emotions; she communicates sadness non-verbally too; discussion of treatment is delayed until after discussion about emotional and practical support. But do these behaviours make the doctor's communication 'excellent', as is claimed? Viewed, instead, from the perspective presented in this Element, the doctor's stance can be questioned. Does she offer a 'secure base' (Section 3)? Does she help the patient be hopeful (Section 6) or does she communicate hopelessness? Do her psychosocial questions inform the consultation? Does it help the patient that she communicates sorrow and unhappiness?

Box 9 Breaking the bad news of cancer diagnosis

This page from Healthtalk (https://healthtalk.org/experiences/bowel-can cer/breaking-news/) collates several patients' experience of diagnosis of bowel cancer. In the second interview, a lady recounts how her surgeon telling her that 'We have a problem' helped her see him as a secure base. By contrast, other interviews recount patients who felt abandoned, misin-formed (about diagnosis or in preparation for diagnostic tests), or disres-pected (being told only after the consultant had explained aspects of the result to accompanying medical students or being told while still undressed).

way in which ethical and scientific perspectives are confounded in this field [205]. Communication skill educators typically appeal to scientific justification of effectiveness when they refer to evidence that training 'improves' skills, and the appearance that CST is scientifically justified has perhaps deterred ethical challenge. Conversely, the belief that CST is inherently important and morally unassailable might explain why its scientific scrutiny has not reached the levels of rigour that are now standard across clinical medicine [251].

For instance, evaluations of CST typically fail to specify the primary out-come variable, instead testing several outcomes. One seminal study included eight outcome measures (counts of different communication skills, each ana-lysed in multiple ways). Although only half showed effects significant at $p<.05$, the authors concluded that training was successful [225] (Moreover, their later conclusion that improvements were maintained at one-year follow-up was based, incorrectly, on not rejecting the null hypothesis of no deterioration rather than on rejecting a null hypothesis of deterioration [226].) In a more recent evaluation that the authors entitled 'rigorous', the main research question was assessed with over 100 separate outcomes of which, again, only around half showed effects favouring training [252]. In areas of clinical medicine that take evaluation more seriously, primary outcomes are routinely specified in advance in published or registered protocols. This protects against the risk that authors 'fish' for positive results amongst a large pool of variables, and it avoids the danger that, without statistical compensation for the increased risk of Type 1 errors (false positives) that arises from multiple testing, reported positive findings are random variation. Multiple outcomes present another problem. It is rarely stated how many, or which ones, should be significant for the training to be regarded as successful. In the studies cited previously, the authors clearly regarded around half as sufficient. But should half be sufficient? And does it matter that, for example, 'empathy' improved but 'checking understanding' did not [225]? Would the opposite result have been just as good (or poor)? The problem here is the absence of a theoretical rationale that allows evaluators to make specific predictions. Similarly, most evaluations report 'improvements' in outcome measures. But few emulate evaluations of interventions in clinical medicine by specifying in advance the *level* of change that would be clinically significant (for a notable exception, see [253]). In a recent study which included patients' ratings of satisfaction with aspects of doctors' communication as outcomes, baseline satisfaction already exceeded 4.5 on a 5-point scale for many ratings, so was probably adequate at the start [252]. Baseline measures of skills are hard to interpret because communication skills literature provides few benchmarks for adequate levels. Therefore, instead of specifying clinically significant changes in advance, communication skills trialists typically aim simply to increase skill performance from the starting level. This implicitly assumes that 'the more the better'. Taken to the limit, the target consultation style would therefore be one filled with talk that displays the measured skills, to the potential exclusion of important clinical tasks. Similarly, in several trials, learners' confidence in their ability to perform learned skills is an outcome measure, e.g. [252,254]; the implicit theory here is that total confidence is better than a level that might leave learners inclined to reflect on their performance (Section 7).

There is another serious problem with quantitative communication research. Its purpose is typically to generalize to a wider population from the sample being studied. For example, the famous finding, from a sample of seventy-four consultations in a US university primary care clinic, that doctors interrupted 69 per cent of patients' opening statements and that the average time of interruption was 18s after patients started speaking [255] is widely cited as showing that 'doctors tend to interrupt patients' opening statements', or that 'doctors interrupt patients after an average of 18s'. However, generalization relies on sampling principles that are hard to achieve in clinical communication. Researchers can rarely sample randomly from the population to which they hope to generalize; as in this instance, samples usually arise from a specific country, city and clinic. Moreover, clinical communication is sensitive to cultural changes so generalizability over time cannot be assumed, whereas findings typically are published a year or more after they are made and are cited after even longer intervals. This is not to argue that quantitative methods have no place in clinical communication research. Rather, we need to be very clear about what they can and cannot achieve, a question which we address in Section 7.

5.5 Conclusion

Assumptions and practices that have become 'taken-for-granted' in CST and its evaluation reflect advocates' commitment to helping practitioners communicate holistically with patients; but they also reflect a climate which has protected those assumptions and practices from robust scientific challenge. When examined critically, the view that good communication depends on deploying skills that are objectively definable – and teachable – is hard to sustain. Once again, we see that the deontological approach that locates quality of communication in reproducible behaviours cannot alone ensure quality. Neither can a consequentialist perspective offer appreciable support for the value of teaching the structured protocols or scripted skills that we have examined in this section. In Section 7, we return to the topic of CST from the perspective that quality of communication depends, not so much on the ability to reproduce skills as on good judgement about when and how to use them. That is, our analysis points again to a virtue ethics perspective; good communication relies on practitioners having the knowledge and motives that allow them to adapt communication flexibly to the needs of individual patients at specific moments in the consultation [6].

6 Communication in Cancer Care

Previous sections introduced influences that have shaped the field of clinical communication. Here, we examine how they play out in one clinical speciality. There are several reasons for choosing cancer care as our 'case study'. First, it has been very significant for communication teachers and researchers as the clinical specialty that has led taking clinical communication seriously, hosting research and developing and supporting communication training programmes. Second, the reality or threat of cancer focuses poignantly the vulnerability that is the key to understanding the patient experience [62]. Third, although often still feared as a fatal disease, survival is steadily improving, and cancer now has elements of a chronic condition, not only an acute one, as people manage their illness or its consequences over time. Therefore, lessons learned from research into communication in cancer care are likely to have wide applicability to other acute and long-term conditions.

6.1 The Emotional Challenge of Cancer

The experience of cancer exemplifies well the biopsychosocial model in extending far beyond the physical dimensions of the disease. Patients with cancer, like those with other physical diseases, are more likely to be depressed or anxious than are healthy members of the normal population. Prevalence figures depend on the assessment procedure and population studied but, in general, 'clinical' levels of depression or anxiety are found in around 15–25 per cent of people treated for cancer [256–258]; post-traumatic stress disorder is present in 5–25 per cent [259]. Fatigue is also common, affecting a third to a half of patients or survivors, with prevalence increasing in more advanced cancers [260,261]. While fatigue is often a direct result of treatments, particularly chemotherapy and radiotherapy, it can also have an emotional or motivational component [261,262].

Physiological mechanisms might link emotional distress to cancer [263,264]. However, there are also obvious psychological reasons why cancer should be distressing. There is the sheer burden of illness and treatment: experiencing pain or discomfort, coping with restrictions on life, managing disclosures of illness to friends and family, and learning to navigate a complex healthcare system in which many different professionals and clinics can be involved. Some patients also feel ashamed of cancer or blame themselves for it or for their 'failure' to cope with it. Cancer can re-evoke previous life traumas; women with breast cancer who recalled being abused as children were more likely than others to be distressed, to feel ashamed of their disease and to blame themselves for it [265]. There is also an existential threat: the 'biographical disruption' that interrupts the expectations that we have for the future, and that signals the prospect of death [266]. Denying the reality or extent of the threat associated with cancer offers some emotional protection, and the tension between denial and the need to learn to accept the illness and its implications can itself be a source of distress [267].

On this analysis, therefore, distress is a normal part of psychological adjustment to cancer, and we should be wary of medicalizing it as a pathology to be treated. Nevertheless, distress can be damaging. Depression, in particular, is associated with poorer treatment adherence and poorer prognosis [268–270]. It also seems that patients with cancer or other physical illnesses who are depressed or anxious use more health service resources, and so cost more to look after [271,272]. Clearly, patients with cancer can have intense emotional needs that practitioners must address along with the cancer itself.

6.2 Attachment in Clinical Relationships in Cancer Care

In health policy and guidance documents and in professional publications we see the assumptions introduced in previous sections about how practitioners should address cancer patients' emotional needs; in particular, that they should use emotional talk to build clinical relationships and provide emotional support [50,273–275]. Over recent years, the expectations on practitioners around emotional support have extended to include identifying patients who are distressed at a 'clinical' level and therefore need additional help. Distress has even been described as patients' '6th vital sign', after temperature, respiration, heart rate, blood pressure and pain [276]. Cancer services are therefore now widely encouraged or mandated to screen patients regularly for depression and anxiety [277,278], although the validity of this practice has been questioned [279,280]. Policy and professional guidance in cancer care also illustrates the second big theme that we have seen in the clinical communication field: practitioners should seek to empower patients by giving them information and involving them in choices over treatment decisions [273,274].

There is a paradox in this guidance; it depicts patients as emotionally vulnerable and needing their practitioners' support, while being sufficiently robust to assimilate clinical information and make treatment decisions. This apparent contradiction arises from the way that the biopsychosocial model has shaped expectations on practitioners (Section 3). Engaging with patients at an emotional level and empowering them to make treatment decisions were both morally inspired ways to humanize clinical practice and respect patients as individuals. Now, however, as we saw in in previous sections, a more evidence-based approach is possible based on understanding more about the nature of clinical relationships.

The theoretical background for understanding findings to be described in this section is the attachment perspective on clinical relationships introduced in Section 3; patients' sense of relationship can arise out of attachment needs rather than being built by practitioners' use of communication skills to engage empathically with patients. A study of newly diagnosed breast cancer patients illustrated how quickly this process can operate in the cancer clinic, without appreciable emotional talk [281]. These patients had just seen their breast surgeon for the first time, after several hours in a rapid diagnosis clinic, in a consultation of around 20 minutes that focused on diagnosis and treatment planning. Before leaving the clinic, patients completed a questionnaire that measures the strength of the alliance patients feel they have with their practitioner, and that previously had mostly been used in counselling or psychotherapy settings – typically after many weeks or months of weekly talk about emotions and feelings. Even after such a brief, clinically focused, interaction, these newly diagnosed patients rated their alliance with their surgeon as stronger than in almost all the published reports in which patients had rated their alliance with psychological practitioners.

Of course, such a relationship does not emerge from patients' attachment needs irrespective of practitioners' behaviour. For patients to feel they have a 'secure base', they need to see practitioners as having the expertise, authority and conscientiousness to provide the security the patient needs [73]; even endorsements of practitioners' expertise by other staff or patients can help

[73,221]. Because attachment figures are not substitutable, continuity of care by the same practitioner is also important [74]. However, cancer clinics are often organized so that patients see different practitioners each time they attend. There is some evidence that a well-functioning clinic can act as a secure base in its own right, but this depends on effective and timely communication between the component parts; without this, patients can feel lost, with nothing to 'hold on to', and lacking confidence in their care [282,283] (Box 10). Conversely, knowing that a single senior clinician oversees their care and is available to them can be comforting, whether or not patients take advantage of that availability [221,244].

In complex clinical care such as for cancer, patients are inevitably sometimes confronted by confusing situations or apparent failures in communication or in the care system. Often patients or, when patients are children, their parents can compensate in actively constructing their 'secure base'. Individual practitioners' abruptness might be attributed, for example, to their being stressed, or perhaps to their knowing what their patients need even better than the patients do [73]. In paediatric cancer care, parents could often 'contain' problems arising in the functioning of the wider team by attributing them to causes, such as work pressure or the demands of healthcare bureaucracy, that protected their need to see the senior clinician as a secure base [73,284]. This is, of course, not to justify failures in care and communication on the grounds that patients or family might find a way to 'contain' them emotionally.

In constructing their secure base, patients or family have further challenges that require mental ingenuity and effort. Being bounded by the constraints of

---

BOX 10 SOURCES OF HOPE AND SECURITY IN CANCER CARE

Many different professions can be involved in cancer care. On Healthtalk, this husband (https://healthtalk.org/pancreatic-cancer/simon-interview-26) describes his experiences of hospital and community care for his wife who had incurable cancer. Two potential sources of a 'secure base' seem to have eluded him: the consultant and the clinical team. In the fourth and sixth extracts, he recounts the shock of diagnosis, and wonders whether the consultant might have 'softened the blow' by giving information more gradually and respecting his wife's wish to retain some hope. In the fifth extract, he describes the apparent lack of coordination amongst the practitioners involved. By contrast, in the eighth extract, he describes finding a secure base in the community nurses, based on their attentiveness, conscientiousness and availability.

a professional relationship, clinical relationships necessarily diverge from attachments in everyday life. Practitioners cannot be burdened with emotions of affection or grief that would be natural within family and social relationships; similarly, patients' entitlement to practitioners' time and support cannot extend beyond their professional role. In breast cancer patients' consultations with surgeons, both parties worked to create a relationship that was authentically personal and intimate, while being firmly circumscribed by professional boundaries [221]. Surgeons described keeping their own emotions out of consultations, for example, by avoiding being tearful when they felt sad or never saying they were 'sorry' when giving bad news (Section 5). Conversely, they described deliberately trying to make each patient feel special, even when they did not recognize her, for example by engaging in social talk; that is, they admitted to acting a role. Similarly, patients were aware of the reality of being a *'stranger'* to surgeons who saw *'hundreds and hundreds'* of patients and who could therefore not know them individually. Nevertheless, patients could feel 'special'. As one explained, *'She's [Surgeon] got to make me feel I'm the only one, although she's doing it constantly. But when I'm there, I'm the only person.'* For both parties, therefore, knowing that the surgeon was acting a role was compatible with feeling that the relationship was sincere and authentic. Authenticity lay in patients recognizing surgeons' conscientious execution of their role.

Clinical relationships therefore depend, not just on practitioners' performance of their role, but on patients' capacity to perform their own complementary role, including the necessary attachment work of constructing the 'secure base' and being able to feel 'special' to the practitioner. Some patients will find this easier than others. We saw in Section 3 how the concept of attachment style can help understand heterogeneity in patients' ability to form trusting clinical relationships and in how they need practitioners to help them. Studies in breast cancer patients have shown one way in which such heterogeneity can arise. Patients who recalled being abused as children felt less supported by their practitioners and by other people in general [285,286]. In one study, only a quarter of women recalling abuse completely trusted their surgeon, compared to two thirds of those with no history of abuse; abuse had left them with a negative 'mental model' of themselves; they could not feel fully supported because they did not feel worthy of others' support [287].

6.3 The Role of Inductive Research in Clinical Communication

We have seen in previous sections that much of the evidence-base for 'evidence-based practice' in clinical communication is weak or tangential. The problem arises because the predominant research paradigm has been quantitative and deductive, whereby researchers' theory and assumptions frame the questions they ask and the methods they use to answer them, thereby tending to perpetuate the ways of thinking from which those questions and methods arose. For example, when researchers use communication coding schemes to investigate whether empathic statements correlate with patient satisfaction, they are not immediately exposed to the possibility that other aspects of practitioners' talk are more important than empathic statements. Questionnaire methods share the same problem; they quantify findings about things that a questionnaire asks about, providing few clues to ones that might be more important.

By contrast, inductive research derives insights from detailed observation, constrained as little as possible by researchers' assumptions. Indeed, good inductive research surprises researchers, changing their views. In clinical communication, inductive research generally uses qualitative methods, and the example in Box 11 illustrates their importance. Careful interviewing that allowed participants to go beyond their initial, normative responses showed that interviewees who first said that they 'want to know everything' went on to complain of having been given too much information [247,288]. Of course, qualitative research lacks generalizability. However, we saw in Section 5 that, given the inherent subjectivity and contextual dependence of communication, generalizability even of quantitative findings is more limited than typically assumed. Recall Kleinman's warning (Section 1) in relation to medical ethics that general principles are of limited help to practitioners, and that the main work of ensuring ethical practice takes place in practitioners' judgements about how to interpret and apply those principles in their work [10]. Similarly, it is in their routine interactions with patients that practitioners must learn the 'practical wisdom' of implementing general moral principles in specific cases [8,9]. Therefore, inductive research into the solutions they find is essential so that these can be understood, critiqued and, potentially, learned from; 'practice-based evidence' is the precursor to 'evidence-based practice' [289].

Critical context for communication encompasses not just observable features of a consultation and of the clinical setting and broader culture in which it is embedded, but also participants' subjective world: what each knows, and what each is seeking and experiencing. Therefore, even qualitative research that is confined to observations of communication will be restricted in the inferences that it can support. To understand and evaluate fully any instance of communication, we also need to know the practitioner's aims and the patient's experience. At the least, practitioners and patients could be debriefed as part of an evaluation of practitioners' communication. In more formal research designs, studying three streams of data simultaneously will mean transcending the methodological 'brands' that have been built around specific types of qualitative data [221,290]. For instance, the way in which practitioners and patients

Box 11 THE IMPORTANCE OF QUALITATIVE RESEARCH IN CLINICAL COMMUNICATION

In questionnaire surveys or structured interviews, respondents are apt to provide culturally normative responses – ones that conform to how they *see themselves* rather than necessarily to how they *are*. These examples show how careful interviewing in qualitative research can expose this contrast.

Here, the researcher (R) is interviewing a patient (P) with breast cancer after she saw her surgeon to receive histology results from recent surgery and to plan further treatment. When asked, at the start of the interview, what she wanted to find out from the consultation, she explained:

P   *I want to know everything . . . I want to know the lot. I want to know what my choices are'.*

Later in the interview, when prompted for her experience of the recent consultation, she complained of being given too much information:

P   *There was all this sort of information around it . . . It was a bit overwhelming. He's a doctor, he's doing this all day. I'm only doing it once. He was showing me, you know, the paper-work, the lab results, you know. I don't want to see all that. I just want him to tell me what's going to happen to me . . . Some of the things he said, I didn't understand . . .*
R   *Well, before you went, what did you want to know?*
P   *I just wanted to know I was going to be OK. That's all. And what they were going to do. And when it was going to happen.*

See https://livrepository.liverpool.ac.uk/3179281/ [247]

In a similar interview, this father of a child diagnosed with leukaemia several months earlier asserts:

You want the facts because the facts tell you where she's at . . . I want specifics, I want to know the details.

But later in the interview he is clear that he needed something different:

There was a couple of times . . . where I wish [haematologist] had been . . . more enthusiastic about how [child] was progressing . . . but the last couple I've been to . . . he really was enthusiastic . . . He started using words like 'Yes, she's doing brilliantly' and you, it obviously makes you feel better.

See https://theoncologist.onlinelibrary.wiley.com/doi/pdfdirect/ 10.1634/theoncologist.2011-0308 [288].

influence each other through their use of speech and language has been studied by discourse analysts or conversation analysts, whereas patients' accounts of their experiences of healthcare have typically lent themselves to thematic or phenomenological approaches. Of course, practical constraints of resources, skills or access often limit researchers to only one type of data or one methodological perspective. However, where the aim is to evaluate communication, researchers need to understand that inferences drawn from only one type of data will be conditional on what is known or unknown from the missing perspectives [290].

In the rest of this section, we see how qualitative research that has become available over the last two decades, and particularly research that has integrated observer, practitioner and patient perspectives, has identified ways in which practitioners and their patients have implemented principles around providing emotional support and involving patients. Most of this work has concerned doctors, reflecting the continued emphasis of clinical communication research, and attachment theory warns us not to apply these findings unquestioningly to relationships with other groups of practitioners (Section 3).

6.4 How Can Cancer Practitioners Provide Emotional Support?

As we saw in Section 3, the starting point for deductive research into patients' support needs has been the principle that practitioners should engage with patients at an explicitly emotional level. By contrast, inductive, qualitative research has begun to illuminate the complexity of practitioners' task in providing support in the context of an asymmetric clinical relationship.

In a detailed study of clinical consultations of parents of children being treated for leukaemia we audio-recorded and analysed dialogue between parents and haematologists, but we also interviewed both parties to the consultation to identify what they wanted – and experienced – from consultations [57,71,86,288]. The parents were emotionally needy, devastated by the fear of losing a child. However, the haematologists wanted to keep their distance and remain objective, and not to engage at an emotional level with the parents. Consultations therefore contained little talk about anything other than clinical results and treatment. However, subsequent interviews with the parents showed that those consultations had comforted them emotionally; comfort came from haematologists being conscientious and authoritative in their clinical care and dialogue with parents. This finding was so striking that we asked parents directly whether they would want to talk to their child's doctor about their fears and feelings. Their response was a clear 'no'. From an attachment perspective, this is unsurprising; in the context of their acute sense of vulnerability, emotional comfort arose from conscientious clinical care.

Moreover, given the emotional turmoil associated with diagnosis of cancer, parents needed practitioners who responded to their distress by remaining rational and *unemotional* [71]. These findings warn us not to regard emotional cues necessarily as pleas for overtly empathic responses, or doctors' failure to provide such responses as always indicating failure of empathy. Emotion can communicate instrumental needs, and doctors' feelings of empathy with patients could therefore be manifest in instrumental responses that address those needs [58,208,221]. It is salutary that, in a sample of cancer patients attending community care who were emotionally distressed, more wanted to speak with a dietician than with a psychologist or social worker [291]!

Patients and parents can actively collaborate in constraining dialogue in consultations to clinical matters, preferring not to introduce psychosocial issues into consultations with practitioners responsible for clinical care [282]. Where clinical teams include a specialist nurse, patients or family can prefer to direct psychosocial problems to them [71,221]. Indeed, many cancer teams make this arrangement explicit. Consistent with this division of responsibilities, there is some evidence that nurses and oncologists see their supportive roles as needing very different communication strategies; oncologists emphasize talk about clinical care while nurses describe relying on overtly psychosocial engagement [86].

Collaboration on constraining what is openly discussed can, of course, signify collusion, whereby patients and practitioners avoid consciously addressing issues, such as those associated with mortality, that present intolerable emotional challenges to both parties [238,240]. Collusion is a risk when practitioners' judgements about when to collaborate with patients' wish to constrain what is voiced in consultation reflect their own emotional needs and values, for instance concerning death [292,293], so practitioners need to become aware of how their own psychology might shape their communication [55,239]. Observation of consultations in patients with advanced cancer, and patients' own accounts, have identified oncologists' practices that might be collusive in avoiding emotionally challenging subjects such as death and dying [209,294,295]. However, the line between collaboration and collusion is hard to define, and future research will need to explore the practitioners' and patients' perspectives also.

Another manifestation of the pervasive assumption that emotional distress in cancer care necessarily indicates emotional needs that must be addressed at an emotional level is the priority currently placed on screening for distress throughout the treatment trajectory [277,296]. Enthusiasm for psychological screening in cancer probably owes much to the analogy with biomedical screening, such as routine mammography to detect breast cancer. However, whereas biomedical screening reveals something otherwise hidden from the patient, psychological screening that relies on responses to transparent questionnaire items can hardly reveal feelings or thoughts of which the patient is unaware [297]. Moreover, screening does not, alone, consistently identify patients who want psychological help [280,297,298]. When patients who screen positive for emotional distress are asked if they want such help, around half or more say 'no' in some studies. Conversely up to a half of those in whom screening identifies no distress do want help. Stigma associated with psychological intervention might explain some distressed patients' reluctance to seek help, and some who are seriously depressed or anxious might not appreciate that services exist to help them. However, a qualitative study indicated another reason [299]. Soon after diagnosis, patients did not want specialist psychological support to help cope with their feelings. Rather, they were coping by focusing on treatment. It was only later in the treatment trajectory that patients were more comfortable engaging with formal emotional support. Once again, we see that, from patients' perspective, clinical management and emotional support are not distinct. Unlike a positive finding from mammography screening, the significance of a positive screen for distress is highly contextual. The challenge for practitioners and services is therefore to help patients identify when they need help, but also to spot those who are not ready to ask but who are 'stuck' in their distress or whose distress is damaging them, for example by reducing adherence to treatment [279,280].

6.5 How Can Cancer Practitioners Manage Information and Involvement

We saw in Section 2 that guidance for practitioners to give 'as much information as possible', or 'the information that the patient wants to have', is unhelpful in practice. Information is essentially infinite and comprises many different types, from disease biology to treatment side effects, and patients cannot make informed decisions about what information they want until they know what the available information shows. Inductive, qualitative research has shown, instead, that patients need practitioners to *manage* information for them carefully, rather than *provide* it and, moreover, that they value knowing that information is being managed for them [282,300]. However, like clinical aspects of cancer care, managing information is complex, given its many functions and consequences for patients and their families.

6.5.1 Information and Hope

The primary need that emerges from patients' own accounts is to have information that is honest, while helping them be positive and hopeful

[62,73,247,282,301–304]. Indeed, patients (and the parents of child patients) are explicit about the asymmetry in their desire for information – wanting to be told good news, while often wanting to be protected from devastating news [73,247,282,288]. They can use cognitive strategies to preserve hope in the face of the fear or reality of poor prognosis [302,305]; for example, comparing themselves to others in a worse situation, or taking comfort from feeling physically well, from starting treatment, or from knowing of other people who have recovered. Therefore being hopeful is not a passive response to a threat, but relies on active 'hope work' [302,305,306] and can take time to learn [288]. Crucially, being hopeful and positive does not mean being unaware of reality. Salander showed how patients can be simultaneously hopeful to the extent of making plans for a future that probably will not exist while knowing the reality of their illness and its implications [302]; he therefore referred to patients 'disavowing' their illness rather than 'denying' it [307,308]. Hope work is, however, interactional as much as cognitive, and practitioners have a crucial role [62,288].

To understand practitioners' role in reconciling honesty with hope, we need to understand more about the nature of hope. In day-to-day language, hope means positive expectations for the future – we 'hope for' something good. However, in the context of the mortal threat of cancer, references to hope can signify keeping positive by *not* thinking about the future, focusing instead on the short-term, even day-to-day. Salander described how engagement in routines and rituals associated with everyday life helps patients distance themselves from the reality of a shortened future [309,310]. Even when the constraints of illness and treatment preclude return to previous routines, patients can find solace in constructing a 'new normality' [311]. In our study of parents of children with leukaemia, parents needed to be positive and hopeful to function effectively in the face of the threat of losing their child, and all wanted the oncologists to help them be hopeful [288]. For these parents, hope meant looking just days or weeks ahead rather than years, but to be able to do this they needed to trust oncologists to take responsibility for the long-term: the child's survival. Faith in the oncologist allowed parents to set aside, rather than deny, their own fears for the future; they needed oncologists to protect them from information about longer-term uncertainties while being positive in providing information about short-term progress. Similarly, adult cancer patients described how trusting their clinical teams to take responsibility for decisions about the future, and the treatment that might grant them a future, allowed them to focus on the present [282,304]. It follows that being hopeful is difficult for patients or parents who cannot fully trust the oncologist, for example because of their experience of previous caring relationships (Section 3).

Patients' need for information that is honest while allowing them to be hopeful clearly presents practitioners with a conundrum, but qualitative research has begun to identify several strategies whereby practitioners 'manage' information to meet this challenge.

Personalizing Information and Responding to Patient Cues

In several studies, oncologists describe making information personal for the patient. For instance, they report managing information-giving by being sensitive to patient cues moment-to-moment, extending or staging information depending on how the patient is responding [239]. A pancreatic cancer surgeon described eschewing printed information leaflets as *'impersonal'*, choosing instead to give patients *'handcrafted'* diagrams that he drew in front of them [312]. A patient who had received such a diagram told the researcher that *'I have that piece of paper . . . You trust your surgeon, or you don't. I trusted him. I knew he'll have done a good job'*. That is, information helped the patient trust the practitioner giving it because it was personalized and given as part of the relationship. As a surgeon in another study explained *'They will remember whether you were kind but they won't remember the words that you've* said' [303]. Similarly, a patient can appreciate an oncologist turning her computer screen towards him to show information, even if he does not understand or remember what that information showed [282].

Just as personalizing information can help support the clinical relationship, the relationship itself helps patients trust the information received. Therefore, when patients want more information than they have received, it can be a sign of lack of trust in the practitioner, that is, that something is wrong in the relationship [32,300]. Failures of care-giving in earlier life or in more recent healthcare can impair the ability to trust (Section 3); or patients or family can have their own specialist knowledge that makes it hard to cede responsibility to practitioners [282,288]. Therefore, while practitioners need to provide the information that such patients explicitly seek, they also need to address patients' implicit needs in relation to a trusting clinical relationship. Doctors who have become patients offer poignant accounts of their role reversal. Paul Kalanithi was an American neurologist who described his experience of lung cancer. Soon after diagnosis he pressed his own doctor for detailed information, including survival probabilities. He later realized that his doctor was right to resist these requests. His desire for information could not be assuaged by information; more information only increased his need, like *'trying to quench thirst with salt water'*. Instead, he needed to be helped to trust his oncologist [313].

Using Different 'Channels' of Information Strategically

Communication literature and guidance typically refer to information as a quantity on a unidimensional scale: patients should have 'full information' or 'as much as they want'. A more complex picture emerged from our qualitative study of how surgeons gave clinical information to breast cancer patients consulting for histology results and treatment planning after surgery to remove their tumours [247]. Surgeons used different 'channels' of information strategically, suggesting the analogy of a spectrum. At the 'short wavelength' end were the biomedical facts that all surgeons gave to every patient. At progressively longer 'wavelengths', surgeons added the kinds of information that allowed patients to build hope. First, they routinely gave information about the next stages in treatment. At a longer 'wavelength' still, they added explicitly evaluative information, like labelling results as 'good'. At the longest 'wavelength', they provided non-verbal cues to the positivity of their message, such as in smiling or tone of voice. Crucially, the surgeons only used the longer wavelength channels when there was something that they could honestly be positive about. That is, although often labelling news as 'good', or explaining how a patient's results were 'better' than they might have been, they never referred to indications of poorer prognosis as 'bad news' or told a patient that the disease was 'worse' than it might have been. Indeed, they were explicit that, contrary to guidance that we saw in Section 5 around breaking bad news, they would never frame information as 'bad' or say they were 'sorry' to give it [247,248]. That is, they were being 'asymmetric' in how they communicated – always giving the key facts and information about further care, and supporting hope where they could, while avoiding messages that could damage patients' capacity to hope. Box 12 illustrates how a patient can complain of having 'no information', when he recalls receiving nothing beyond the 'shortest wavelength' biomedical facts.

Using Linguistic Conventions for Positivity

Everyday language contains conventions to manage listeners' morale. Popular exhortations to 'keep positive' or to 'look on the positive side' are usually unhelpful in a cancer context because the implied obligation to conceal distress can add to the burden that patients or families feel [295,314]. However, observations of consultations with oncologists showed that they drew on another linguistic strategy for conveying information truthfully but positively [315]. Potentially negative clinical facts in the context of treatment planning were typically followed by more positive information; for example '*yours is potentially serious, but most of these are cured*'. The significance of the strategy is easily illustrated by imagining the reverse pairing: '*most of these are cured but*

Patients often complain of needing 'more information' than they have been given. Sometimes, this complaint belies problems in the clinical relationship that go beyond information provision. In the first extract from this patient's interview on Healthtalk (https://healthtalk.org/experi ences/prostate-cancer/how-prostate-cancer-affects-you/) he complained of having 'no real information'. But he recounts having received the key information: his diagnosis and uncertain prognosis. What was perhaps missing was information in the other 'channels' beyond biomedical facts. Because that was missing, he seems to have felt abandoned and hopeless.

yours is potentially serious'. The same information would be given, but in a way that would make hope more difficult.

6.5.2 Information and Involvement

Receiving information is classically depicted in clinical communication literature as the precursor to making decisions about treatment or care. Cancer care can sometimes present patients with decisions that practitioners cannot or do not lead, for instance where there is equipoise between treatment options or where they are offered entry to clinical trials. There are also patients who, because of their own experience or knowledge, cannot, or do not want to, delegate decisions to practitioners. And practitioners must give information that satisfies medicolegal requirements for informed consent. However, in general, we saw in Section 2 that the assumption that patients routinely seek information to make treatment decisions is based on a view of individual autonomy that poorly fits the reality of clinical care, in which patients typically look to practitioners to lead treatment decisions. Unsurprisingly, therefore, inductive research into how decisions in cancer care are made in practice shows a role for information in decision-making that is very different from the prevailing concept of informed choice. Although not a formal research study, one of the earliest published accounts of a patient's perspective on decision-making in cancer was a personal reflection by an eminent doctor who became a patient. Ingelfinger described painful indecision when doctors sought his views on treatment of his own cancer [316]. He found relief only after following a friend's advice to consult a doctor whom he could trust to take responsibility for decisions. As we saw earlier, entrusting the longer-term to practitioners allows patients to find hope by focusing on the short-term.

Qualitative evidence bears out Ingelfinger's experience; patients described needing to trust practitioners to take responsibility for decisions [41,73,304]. But receiving information can help patients take ownership of those decisions. For instance, in a UK breast cancer service, surgeons did not usually offer treatment options for patients to choose between when they returned to the clinic for histology results after surgery. Instead, based on recommendations from the multidisciplinary team, surgeons routinely told patients what the treatment would be [41]. But they also provided reasons to justify their decisions, and having that information helped patients to take ownership of them – feeling committed to them as the right ones (Box 13). A few patients were, however, unconvinced, with worries that surgeons had not addressed. It seems that the surgeons had a 'script' that satisfied most patients, but left insufficient opportunity for those with concerns to raise them. The solution would be a simple modification to the script; the surgeons could prompt patients for their reaction to, and concerns about, what they had proposed.

Information needs in relation to treatment decisions cannot therefore be separated from the role of information to support hope and trust, and neither function can be understood except in the context of the clinical relationship [32,62]. Patients' need for hope means being able to trust practitioners to be sufficiently expert and conscientious to take responsibility for decisions about care, and practitioners' management of information is central in this process. Similarly, the management of information at the level of the clinical team can determine patients' ability to see the team as a secure base; unclear, inconsistent or inaccurate information can leave patients feeling confused and alone rather than secure in practitioners' care [283] (Box 10).

6.6 Conclusion

In this section, we have drawn heavily on inductive research in which practitioners and patients agreed to cooperate with social scientists, to be interviewed by them and to have their discussions recorded and observed. Many practitioners will be cautious about research into their communication, particularly given the criticism they receive from communication researchers and educators. Therefore, those willing to open their consultations to researchers' scrutiny are a selected subgroup, and the communication strategies that this section described might not be widespread. Conversely, there are probably many

Box 13 'Owning' decisions without making them

When breast cancer patients saw their surgeon post-operatively for histology results and planning of further treatment, the surgeons typically told patients what the next treatment would be. But they gave reasons, and these allowed patients to 'own' the decisions, as this patient illustrates.

> *They put it straight to me, a mastectomy. [Surgeon] did say that they could have just removed the part where the cancer was. But ... it was almost certain, she said, 'You'll have to come back and have further operations ... Unless we're certain we've got every bit of it, we'd rather take the whole thing away and then we know we've got everything.'*

In this consultation, the surgeon (S) reported histology results, then told the patient (P) what treatment will be:

S *In this situation what will we do next? First thing will be radiotherapy. We did discuss that. Since we are removing a little bit of breast you may need extra treatment for the rest of the breast just to, you know, reduce the chance of coming back.*

P *Yeah.*

S *That is the radiotherapy.*

P *Right.*

S *For that you will be seeing one of the oncologists.*

Interviewed after the consultation, the patient and her husband (H, present in the consultation) illustrate how the surgeon's approach instilled confidence.

P *Three weeks of radiotherapy and tablets for five years and regular mammogram every 12 months. I thought it was excellent ... There was nothing really that I needed to ask him really, because he was thorough ...*

H *He was confident right from the word go which made us feel confident about it.*

See https://livrepository.liverpool.ac.uk/3179287/ [41]

more strategies awaiting exposure by future inductive research. However, the point of such research is not to describe what routinely happens, but to identify strategies in use, examine them critically, and make them known so that other researchers, educators and, ultimately, practitioners can learn from them.

7 Towards the Next Generation of Communication Teaching

In Section 5, we saw how communication skills teaching (CST), like other technologies in clinical communication, had sought to implement the biopsychosocial model of care: practitioners should be concerned with the psychological and social dimensions of illness, and their care should extend beyond the biology of the disease to a holistic concern with the psychosocial needs that surround it. We also saw that CST had taken shape when there was still little detailed observational evidence about how the psychological needs associated with physical disease arise and are addressed or thwarted in consultations. The next generation of communication education for practitioners can be informed by the inductive evidence that has become available, by the advances in ethical thinking and psychological theory described in previous sections and by the accumulating evidence of the outcomes of the current generation of CST. Like any educational initiative, it can also be informed by educational theory, or pedagogy.

7.1 Pedagogy for Clinical Communication Teaching

7.1.1 Educational Pedagogy: A Framework for Setting Objectives

First published in 1956 but revised subsequently [317–319], Bloom's 'taxonomy of educational objectives' is still widely used in education to help craft learning objectives tailored to the subject (Box 14). It prompts educators, first, to distinguish three distinct domains in which they might create objectives: behavioural actions, or skills; knowledge and cognition; and affect, or emotion, including the attitudes and values that underlie emotional reactions. For each domain, Bloom's framework further prompts educators to decide the *level* of change to be sought in learners, from very limited levels through progressively more complex ones that demand more of both learners and educators. The domain of knowledge and cognition has received most attention from educationists, but each domain is potentially relevant to clinical communication.

The Behavioural Action Domain

As we saw in Section 5, the term 'skill' has been applied widely to diverse aspects of clinical communication, such as 'appropriate eye contact' or

Box 14 Bloom's taxonomy of educational objectives

Educators can create learning objectives in each of three domains and, within each domain, at progressively more complex levels [317-319]. (See https://www.simplypsychology.org/blooms-taxonomy.html#Cognitive-Domain-1956.)

'empathy', which defy behavioural definition. Nevertheless, potentially important objectives for clinical communication might be created in this domain, where learners need to learn behavioural repertoires that they might not have acquired before clinical training. At the lowest levels, objectives would be simple scripted behaviours such as checking a patient's identity to start a consultation. At more complex levels, they would encompass interactive skills, which cannot be fully scripted because they depend on patients' responses; for example, organizing, signposting and sequencing information, or 'de-escalation' protocols to respond to challenging patients. Learning specific frameworks to structure or sequence a consultation, like SPIKES (Section 5), might be valuable for new practitioners, or ones in training, who lack the experience to improvise. Learning linguistic techniques of argumentation could help doctors lead patients' decision-making (Section 4) [320–322]. However, given the unpredictability of conversation with another individual, high-level objectives in this domain will emphasize, not the performance of reproducible skills, but learners' flexibility and creativity in adapting them to individual patients and situations [6,206].

The Affective, or Emotional, Domain

While CST places a high priority on patients' emotions, and on practitioner–patient dialogue at an emotional level, it has less to say about whether and how educators can engage with practitioners' own character and emotional experience [6]. By contrast, the analysis in this Element has pointed repeatedly to the need to recognize that quality of clinical communication depends on practitioners' character and motives. Therefore, there is much scope for creating objectives in this domain. At the basic level, learners need to be aware of their values and emotions in communication with patients [56,192]. At higher levels of complexity, they will be able to question and, where necessary, modify these. At the highest, they will evolve a value system that reflects their own individual character and experience as well as the demands of their profession [248].

The Knowledge and Cognition Domain

Surprisingly, CST has not emphasized learning objectives in the knowledge domain, in striking contrast with other clinical subjects, like physiology or pharmacology, in which learners acquire a sound knowledge base before deploying relevant skills. For instance, even after two decades during which its relevance to clinical practice has been described [49,82,323], attachment theory is missing from major textbooks on clinical communication [324]. Other relevant areas of knowledge are also absent from communication textbooks and curricula. Without being taught about the psychological effects of the fear or reality of serious disease it will be harder for practitioners to understand their patients' experience and to judge how best to support them [6]. Similarly, practitioners will need to know how patients explain, or make sense of, illness so that they can craft explanations that find common ground between biomedical and lay knowledge systems [325]. Educators could also disseminate knowledge of communication strategies that inductive research has discovered practitioners using, such as those in Section 6. Without a strong knowledge base, learners are placed in the role of technicians rather than scientifically grounded practitioners; that is, following rules without the understanding that would allow them to make good judgements about when and how to apply – and, where necessary, break – those rules.

At the lowest levels in this domain, educators' objectives will be for learners simply to remember what they have been taught, perhaps reproducing it for written exams. Therefore, didactic, classroom teaching will be important, just as for other clinical subjects. At progressively more complex levels, objectives will be for learners to evaluate knowledge critically, and to be creative and imaginative in how they use it to make judgements in specific situations with specific patients. That practitioners are curious about their patients will be an objective, too, so they can learn from them.

The knowledge and cognition domain prompts educators to look beyond the kinds of knowledge that allow judgements only about abstract or technical matters. Dating from Aristotle's accounts of the virtues that underlie good judgement, the concept of 'practical wisdom' refers to knowing how to make judgements that are sensitive to the nature and circumstances of specific situations. In the present context, it means the practical know-how whereby practitioners with good motivations weigh up what goals are important in any clinical interaction and judge how to achieve them; that is, to do the right thing at a specific moment with a specific patient [9,326]. It therefore depends, not just on having the right motives and knowledge, but on the experience of working with these in practice [210,327].

In each domain, therefore, we see that the highest levels of learning emphasize creativity and originality. Several educationists and researchers in clinical communication have already argued that the quality of communication depends on these levels of learning; that is, not so much on practitioners' ability to reproduce skills as on their good judgements about when and how to use them, and on their ability to be creative and imaginative in adapting to the unpredictability of clinical practice[56,192,206,228,328]. Experienced educators will already work towards those higher-level objectives, particularly when they meet with experienced practitioners. However, to the extent that the scientific and educational literature that informs CST neglects this level of objective it will not inform their work, which will therefore remain a type of 'craft' learned through experience or passed on from one teacher to another.

7.1.2 Pedagogy in Creative Arts: Ambiguity and Creativity

The emphasis on reproducible behavioural skills in clinical communication literature perhaps reflects the continued influence of a scientifically oriented pedagogy, which seeks reproducibility and certainty in learning outcomes based on generalized rules. By contrast, pedagogy associated with creative arts recognizes that the inherent uncertainty of creative work is the space within which learners experiment and improvise [224,329–331]. Langewitz therefore advocated using '*more colourful and less deterministic language*', being more '*poetic and less prosaic*', in presenting communication to learners [176]. Were communication educators to draw on objectives and approaches more familiar in creative arts, they would primarily aim for learners to make good judgements that, informed by general principles, also reflect the demands and opportunities of the specific context. For example, Eggly [243] proposed that, rather than teach practitioners to anticipate, plan and script consultations about bad news (Section 5), they need help to adapt communication to the informational and emotional needs that arise throughout an interaction. Therefore, from this pedagogical perspective, there would be more emphasis on learning experiences that are less predictable; in particular, more learning with patients in real clinical scenarios would make contextual variability and ambiguity explicit. While the emphasis on reproducibility and uniformity has favoured the use of simulated consultations, some educators and, indeed, students value 'real patient learning' in an apprenticeship approach that more realistically prepares for the variability of clinical practice [332–334]. It is important to acknowledge, once again, that many experienced educators whose teaching is already shaped, not just by the CST literature, but by the demands of learners confronting the reality of clinical care, will already work towards these ends. However, a conceptual framework that encompasses creativity could be more valuable than one based on communication skills in helping them reflect on their work and to describe and develop it.

Pedagogy in creative arts has also had to confront the holistic nature of work that cannot be reduced to components that can be assessed objectively. A painting's quality would not be judged by evaluating the background, then specific objects, before summing the ratings. Educationists in creative arts concern themselves instead with holistic judgements of 'rightness of fit' rather than reductionist algorithms [329]. Just as with the elements of a painting, the quality of any element of communication only exists in its context: the whole clinical situation and the communication surrounding it [176]. Indeed, patients can be more concerned with the whole picture – their impression of practitioners' character and caring – than with specific communication behaviours [73,229]. Nevertheless, in CST, the quality of communication is routinely assessed by aggregating ratings of its components – typically the performance of specific skills or achievement of specific tasks. Global ratings with psychometric properties comparable to those of checklists have long been available to assess clinical communication [335–337]. However, in developing their use further, there is an important lesson from creative pedagogy; the validity of such evaluations accrues less from the assessment's design and psychometric properties than from the selection and scrutiny of the expert assessors who must judge whether the communication 'worked'. Eisner described experts in this context as needing the expertise of 'connoisseurs', arising from intimate engagement with their field [224]. Patients' perspectives are sometimes advocated on the grounds that their subjective experience defines the meaning of communication. In a clinical context, however, meaning depends also on clinical considerations and professionalism. Therefore, assessors will not necessarily be patients, but could include practitioners recognized as good communicators, or researchers with intimate knowledge of the clinical context of the assessment.

Given that the quality of communication depends on the context, and that this context includes each participant's subjective experience and priorities, observers – however expert – will have to make their judgements with incomplete contextual knowledge. Recognizing that assessments will therefore still carry some uncertainty has important implications for educators and researchers. For summative assessments during training, educators will have to identify learners whose communication is unsafe or damaging; however, there is less point in trying to allocate an 'objective' quality score [338]. For researchers evaluating communication in practice, more humility will be needed than is sometimes apparent in the way that they criticize practitioners' communication. After all, in this Element we have seen potentially valuable communication strategies that practitioners have discovered for themselves which were apparently unknown to communication 'experts'.

Finally, pedagogy from creative arts has implications for how educators manage learners' motivation [172,339,340]. Rather than relying on external motivators such as exam passes or quality ratings, there would be a more explicit focus on stimulating, and drawing on, learners' internal motivators; for instance, their valuing of communication, their curiosity about patients and the desire to become more effective practitioners.

7.1.3 Evidence-Based Pedagogy: How Practitioners Learn Communication

A third source of pedagogy arises from evidence about how practitioners naturally learn communication. Communication literature has shown only limited interest in this, despite a long-standing concern with an informal 'hidden curriculum' whereby students and practitioners are assumed to acquire professional and communication habits from those around them in routine practice [326,341]. Nevertheless, studies of how practitioners approach communication and how they learn to communicate could inform formal curriculum design.

First, doctors' communication is probably mostly directed by their goals rather than by communication rules. A recent study examined their use of skills that, according to structured education models should be deployed sequentially: from those for 'initiation', 'gathering information' and 'planning' to ones for 'closing'. In practice, doctors used skills from these different 'stages' flexibly and iteratively instead of sequentially [342]. Similarly, evidence in primary care shows how multiple and often changing goals over the course of a consultation drive GPs moment-to-moment selection of communication strategies [213]. Viewing communication as goal-directed problem-solving potentially offers a more realistic way to engage with practitioners than by focusing on communication skills and structures decontextualized from what the practitioners are trying to achieve [212]. In other reports, doctors' explanations of the importance of experimentation and reflection in learning about communication recall formal accounts in ethical and educational literature of the role of experience and reflection in the acquisition of 'practical wisdom', described earlier in this section [326,327]. In surgery [248] and general practice [343] doctors described observing other practitioners' communication, reflecting on it and choosing strategies selectively to try out and adapt. The endpoint was to have integrated what they had learned into a personal style which reflected their own identity and character and the goals they sought to achieve with their patients. In this way, communication could simultaneously be both learned and authentic [221] (Section 6). The surgeons were critical of CST they had received because it made them feel insincere, as if they were being taught to pretend [248]. This does not mean that they gained nothing from that teaching. However, they had selected and adapted specific approaches or techniques until they felt right for them. This limited evidence base points to the need for future communication teaching, particularly with experienced practitioners, to acknowledge learners' pre-existing expertise and individuality [344]. Rather than 'training' pre-defined ways of communicating, teaching can 'educate', whereby what is learned reflects the active role of the learner as well as the teacher.

7.2 Pointers to the Next Generation of Communication Teaching

A recent consensus statement set the scene for renewing communication teaching in ways that diverge in important respects from the past [192]. It was concerned specifically with cancer care which, as we have seen, has long been in the lead in communication teaching. It revised the consensus of European experts reported ten years earlier [50], advising educators to look beyond standardized skills to the attitudes and emotional feelings that shape practitioners' communication. To help practitioners understand the relational context of communication, educators should teach about relationships but also help learners to achieve and maintain the emotional self-awareness that would help foster effective relationships. Implementing this guidance will clearly need educational methods that go beyond training communication skills, to include fostering the competencies and qualities that inform and motivate their judgements about how to communicate in practice [6]. That is, the current deontological approach will need to give way to one closer to virtue ethics. Reports over recent decades provide some pointers to approaches that go beyond the teaching of skills to engage with learners also at the levels of knowledge and cognition, and emotions and attitudes.

Several reports have focused on empathy, reflecting its central importance in communication literature. Recognizing that practitioners' empathy for their patients should start with understanding them and *feeling* empathic towards them rather than with empathic *behaviours*, some educators have explored narrative and experiential approaches to sensitize learners to patients' experience [345]. In one account of teaching about 'bad news' consultations, junior doctors saw video-recordings of clinical communication informed, unusually, not by assumptions about what patients would value, but by the accounts of patients who had watched those recordings [228]. Reflecting on real or fictional patient narratives or poignant medically related stories from personal experience, popular literature or films has also been advocated as a way to inform empathy in doctors in training or practice [334,346]. Medical students have accompanied patients through a series of medical encounters [326], or have even been hospitalized [347] so that they could reflect on the experience of being a patient. Some educators have suggested that theory about acting could help teach empathy. They argue that teaching skills promotes 'surface acting', whereby learners perform behaviours associated with empathy regardless of whether or not they feel empathic. By contrast, 'deep acting' means learning to feel empathy and responding to that feeling [348,349]; that is, instead of creating a task focus in learners, they could be helped to use their own feelings to become attuned to the 'atmosphere' of a consultation [176]. While actors are widely used in CST to play the part of patients, expertise in acting might inform teaching itself.

When learners are experienced practitioners, they bring their own experience and expertise – and the authority that arises from that experience and expertise. Although experienced communication skills teachers will already draw on that background in teaching sessions, they are not helped by the theoretical underpinning of CST which emphasizes expert-defined skills, giving little status to communication strategies, such as those in Section 6, that practitioners have developed informally [344]. Some educators have described approaches to communication education that explicitly put practitioners' expertise at the centre. Rollnick et al. [344] contrasted traditional 'workshop' training, typically held outside practitioners' place of work and with objectives and content directed by educators, with an approach they called 'context-bound' training that explicitly rejected the assumption that the practitioners lacked skills that they needed experts to teach. To ground training in their learners' (GPs) everyday experience rather than the educators' knowledge of communication skills, training was in the GPs' premises and shaped by their own preferences. Participating GPs consulted with a simulated patient shortly before meeting with colleagues in groups facilitated by the educators. Crucially, each GP received a transcript of their consultation, so that group discussion could be informed by GPs' reflection on their own experience. The educators accepted that, as the experts on what they needed, each GP would take something different from the training. As one GP explained, '*It wasn't about communication skills training. It was about getting better at what we do every day.*'

Expertise is not, though, a 'zero sum', in which the educators need to claim less to make space for that of learners. Some recent reports describe initiatives anchored in practitioners' clinical settings, and in their everyday experience and expertise, in which educators provide specialist knowledge to inform practitioners' own judgements about communication. Stiefel et al. described how individual supervision from a psychological expert could foster oncologists' awareness of ways in which their own personal history and emotional responses complicated their relationships with patients [350,351]. Realistically, resources for individual supervision will be scarce in many services. Therefore a more cost-effective approach could be that described by Salander [237]; the psychological expert facilitated a group of oncology practitioners meeting periodically to analyse communication and relational challenges in their work. As well as using scarce psychological expertise efficiently, this format allowed peers to contribute their own insights to solutions that were clinically realistic for the context. Many communication dilemmas for experienced practitioners in oncology and other specialties contain ethical dilemmas, where the 'right thing' to do or say is unclear. Prompted by emotional and moral challenges created by restrictions associated with the COVID-19 pandemic, Delany et al. [352] described 'reflective ethics discussions', in which the source of external expertise to facilitate reflective groups was bioethics rather than psychology. Delany et al. were explicit that the function of external expertise was not to tell practitioners what to do, but to help practitioners reflect on what they were experiencing so they could find their own responses.

A programme of teaching that the originators called 'Program to Enhance Relational and Communication Skills (PERCS)' [353–356] illustrates how the term 'skills' is now widely used simply to mean 'good communication', because this programme goes far beyond a concern with behavioural skills to include many of the curriculum elements described previously. It starts with an explicit statement of philosophy and pedagogy. This grounds teaching in the uniqueness of clinical encounters and the complexity of clinical practice in which good communication depends, not on reproducible skills, but on practitioners' attitudes, values and relational capacities including curiosity about patients, and in which there is typically no one 'correct' way to communicate [355]. The curriculum format, centred on scenarios played by actors, allows educators to contribute expertise, while eliciting and valuing participants' own expertise and insights. Rather than play standardized patients, the actors improvise so that scenarios replicate the unpredictability of routine practice. Arising from a paediatric setting, PERCS has been extended to other specialties, and has included multiple disciplines and both students and experienced practitioners.

These examples illustrate features that will characterize the next generation of communication education: an emphasis on relational and contextual aspects of communication, recognition of patients' and practitioners' individuality, respect for learners' expertise, and provision for learners to understand and reflect on what they are learning. They also illustrate that, just as there is typically no one way to communicate in any situation, there will be no single way to teach communication; experimentation will be needed. Approaching communication teaching from a perspective closer to virtue ethics than to a deontological emphasis on behavioural skills brings further possibilities. Communication teaching will overlap considerably with teaching of medical ethics and professionalism, which focus explicitly on learner qualities that influence their care of, and communication with, patients [8,345,357]. Therefore, expertise and insights from teaching those subjects can inform communication teaching. For instance, communication skills teachers have long been concerned about limited transfer of skills from teaching settings into clinical practice. However, education that emphasizes learners' qualities will refocus this concern with generalization. Learners need to transfer, not predefined skills, but the ability to adapt communication to the context [358]. An emphasis on the underlying qualities that guide this adaptability – including knowledge, curiosity and conscientiousness – would provide the continuity that is needed between formal teaching and informal practice.

Communication research and teaching can also engage with current debates around virtues and their relationship to practitioners' behaviour, that have been fuelled by disenchantment with the deontological approach of behavioural guidelines and protocols as ways to help clinicians with morally ambiguous judgements in clinical practice [8]. These debates emphasize that, while understanding *why* moral considerations such as patient-centredness are important will be necessary for learners to embrace the principles, or virtues, that should guide their relationships with patients [2], merely talking about virtues will be insufficient; habit-forming practice or observation of skilled practitioners is also necessary [357]. Therefore, there will be much more concern than now with the communication expertise of educators and supervisors. Technical knowledge about communication will be insufficient, and learners will also need exposure to practitioners who are recognized as having acquired the 'practical wisdom' of excellent clinical communicators [8,326]. Social scientists or practitioners who lack clinical experience in the specific clinical context of their learners – for example when psychologists, nurses, GPs or psychiatrists deliver training for cancer clinicians – are therefore necessarily constrained in what they can achieve alone. Ethicists applying virtue ethics ideas to clinical education also warn that merely observing experienced practitioners is insufficient. Learners need to be helped to reflect on what they observe and on their own behaviour [327]. Therefore, for example, observing practices associated with patient centredness could be a stage in the formation of authentically patient-centred practitioners, provided that learners acquire in parallel the capacity for self-reflection through which they can internalize the values of authentic patient-centredness [2]. The authors of one educational program explicitly designed to facilitate practical wisdom in clinical interactions chose to embed their medical students in continuous longitudinal relationships – with patients, peers and senior doctors – in the belief that this would promote real reflection better than more fleeting encounters would [326].

A virtue ethics perspective does not mean seeing practitioners as saintly and infallible, or on trajectories to becoming so. Evidence that human behaviour is heavily determined by situational factors that can outweigh the influence of people's virtues [359] is a warning that the qualities which clinical training will seek to inculcate have to jostle with practitioners' other attributes and priorities, and with the reality of clinical care and professional life. In the present context the value of a virtue ethics perspective is therefore not as a theory about how character might outweigh situational influences [360], but as a pragmatic way to address the reality that good communication relies on practitioners making good judgements for good reasons. Moreover, the capacity to make good judgements is not an end-state to be reached by sufficient training and experience; rather, it is a continued process of learning and reflection [326,359].

7.3 Evaluation of Communication Teaching

7.3.1 What Will Be Evaluated?

These new and experimental approaches will not be evaluated solely by measuring learners' reproduction of skills. The challenge of evaluating communication education therefore returns us to the start of this Element, where we distinguished different philosophical perspectives on evaluating communication itself (Section 1).

Approaching evaluation *deontologically*, educators will want to know whether learners' behaviour has changed in ways that indicate that they can follow pre-defined rules or display taught skills. Student practitioners will need to show that they can check patients' identity; and they might need to show that they have learned frameworks, such as SPIKES (Section 5), to structure consultations before they become sufficiently experienced to acquire flexibility. Teachers of specific techniques such as argumentation or de-escalation of aggression will need to confirm that learners can display the taught techniques. Given that such skills emerge in interaction with patients and that their significance will be highly contextual, evaluators will not be able simply to count the number of times skills are used; assessment will need to be more holistic (Section 5).

There will also continue to be outcomes to assess from a *consequentialist* perspective. At a minimum, educators need to know that learners are positive about training they have received – the starting point for willing participation in future and for gaining employers' funding and support. Many previous evaluations of training have also measured learners' confidence about communication. However, given the need for practitioners to retain sufficient self-criticism that they reflect continually on their communication, this outcome is ambiguous. Educators might evaluate learners' success in completing specific tasks, such as communicating respect or obtaining necessary information, whether from patients' own report or the judgement of expert observers. However, aggregating assessments of a range of such tasks will not alone indicate the quality of the whole consultation, given that practitioners' goals can be many and fluctuating as a consultation proceeds (Section 5); more holistic judgements will be needed. Clearly, the outcomes of ultimate importance concern patients. However, the common use of patient satisfaction risks being misleading; increased satisfaction is no evidence that patients have benefited clinically (Section 4). Ultimately, clinical outcomes are key. Realistically, however, the effects of changes in communication might be detectable only with sample sizes closer to those of epidemiological designs than the small-N studies that are typical in communication research. For instance, associations of primary care patients' symptom improvement with their experience of consultation were detected in a sample of 750 [361], and a meta-analysis that showed that doctors' brief advice could improve smoking cessation included 31,000 patients [362]. Even were such studies to be widely available, clear implications for practitioners would only arise where teaching had narrowly targeted precisely defined behaviours. For most teaching programmes, the contextual nature of communication means that findings would be generalizations, saying little about how the communication being assessed unfolded in specific moments with specific patients.

Given that learners' qualities that motivate and inform their communication will have been targets of curricula in future, educators will need to approach evaluation also from a *virtue ethics* perspective. Just as for other clinical sciences, they will assess whether learners have understood what they have been taught at a level at which they can critique what they know and be creative in applying that knowledge to new situations. However, attitudes, values and qualities such as curiosity, conscientiousness and self-reflection will be more challenging to assess, and evaluators will need to explore new forms of assessment [363].

7.3.2 How Will It Be Evaluated?

Given the prevailing emphasis on quantitative evaluation, many educators will seek to develop questionnaires or rating scales to measure these attitudes, values and qualities. However quantitative evaluation will need much greater methodological discipline than has been typical previously in evaluating CST. If educators perform randomized controlled trials with a view to statistically generalizable inferences, they will need to adopt the rigorous design standards to which clinical trialists are held, and that have mostly been disregarded in evaluations of CST (Section 5). Showing that teaching produces statistically significant changes in learners' behaviour or even patient outcomes by comparison with a control group is not, however, the only – or even the most valuable – approach to evaluation, and such generalized findings are hard to relate to practice [364].

Teachers of biomedical ethics or professionalism are not expected to justify their work by RCTs of its outcomes. Instead, the place of such subjects in the curriculum is based on moral claims to their status as essential elements of patient-centred clinical training. From this perspective, communication educators should not need quantitative outcome evidence to justify inclusion of their own subject in clinical curricula. Evaluation could instead embrace the debate, diversity and innovation that is more characteristic of medical humanities. In this context, quantitative evaluations that lack a primary outcome, or that are under-powered, might still be valuable. They could help refine interventions or prepare for formal outcome studies, but evaluators should not conflate exploratory and definitive evaluation; based on findings from designs that are essentially exploratory, they should not make claims about efficacy (Section 5).

Even used in this way, though, quantitative methods are limited in their value for exploratory research, because they tend to perpetuate the concepts or categories to which outcomes are allocated for quantification. By contrast, in this Element, we have seen how qualitative research can challenge the validity of current assumptions. As we saw in Section 6, qualitative methods allow inductive research; instead of examining communication through the lenses of pre-existing ideas, new implications are drawn from real-life instances of communication. Used in this way, qualitative research recognizes that there is typically no single correct way to communicate in any instance, and that communication can only be understood in its context. Similarly, qualitative evaluation of teaching will recognize that there will be no single way to teach communication [6]. There is a further lesson to be learned from qualitative research into communication itself. Just as such research can respond to the subjectivity and contextual dependence of communication by examining patient and practitioner perspectives as well as the communication between them, evaluation of communication teaching will need to be multidimensional. That is, observations of the teaching process can be informed by accounts of the participating teachers and learners and of patients who participate in the teaching or who consult learners after the teaching.

7.4 Conclusion

While the portrayal of clinical communication as made up of skills perhaps helped facilitate the subject's incorporation into clinical curricula alongside other 'clinical skills', educators and researchers need a richer conceptual background for developing and evaluating the next generation of clinical communication education. This section has pointed to ways for communication education to escape the constraints of the skills model. Doing so will help those educators whose teaching already goes beyond skills to articulate and reflect on what they are doing; and it will help to build the pedagogical base for the next generation of communication education to become as intellectually lively as it should be, given its position at the interface of ethics, theory and practice.

8 Epilogue

This Element has many practical limitations. It has not been a textbook, and has not told the reader how to communicate with specific patients in specific situations. It has disregarded many aspects of clinical communication that challenge practitioners and interest researchers. Its emphasis on cancer care, and on hospital treatment, has been at the expense of attention to long-term conditions or to primary care, and to settings in which patients might act in a more consumerist way, such as aesthetic surgery. It has followed the available data in focusing on doctors, to the neglect of other practitioners. There has been more emphasis on what we can learn from practitioners than on what practitioners get wrong. Arguably, though, it has pointed to the elephant in the room of much previous clinical communication research, education and guidance. Googling 'doctor-patient relationships' or 'doctor-patient communication' and selecting 'images' fills the screen with pictures of interactions between people who are mostly smiling, and in which it would often be hard to identify who is the doctor without the emblematic white coat or stethoscope worn by one party. Often the picture centres on information being happily shared on a computer screen or tablet computer or clipboard. The 'elephant' that these images conceal is patients' vulnerability. Mostly, patients seek medical care because they feel ill, fear that they are ill, or want to avoid being ill: they are suffering, or fear suffering in future. Their fear or discomfort, or their lack of medical training, typically precludes the dispassionate examination of medical information that the images portray. So those images – like much of the communication research and teaching discussed in this Element – present an idealized view of clinical relationships that excludes their defining feature.

The motives for portraying clinical relationships in this unrealistic way can only be guessed at. Perhaps there is unwillingness to confront the realities of morbidity and mortality that lie at the heart of clinical relationships [365]. There are commercial and professional interests in play, too. Communication skills teaching has become big business in universities and healthcare organizations, and the deontological emphasis on teaching expert-defined skills has given those experts, including many non-clinical social scientists, authority and influence over clinical professions. Whatever the reasons, this Element has argued that many patients and practitioners will be poorly served by the view of clinical relationships portrayed in those images and in much of the clinical communication literature. Instead, the Element has offered patients' vulnerability and dependence as a starting point for understanding and guiding clinical relationships. But this *is only* a starting point.

References

1. Street Jr RL, Makoul G, Arora NK, et al. How does communication heal? Pathways linking clinician-patient communication to health outcomes. *Patient Educ Couns* 2009;74(3):295–301.

2. Duggan PS, Geller G, Cooper LA, et al. The moral nature of patient-centeredness: Is it 'just the right thing to do'? *Patient Educ Couns* 2006;62 (2):271–6.

3. Kinmonth AL, Woodcock A, Griffin S, et al. Randomised controlled trial of patient centred care of diabetes in general practice: impact on current well-being and future disease risk. *Br Med J* 1998;317(7167):1202–8.

4. Gauthier CC. Teaching the virtues: Justifications and recommendations. *Camb Q Healthc Ethics* 2009;6(3):339–46. https://doi.org/10.1017/S0963180100008033.

5. Van Norden BW. Virtue ethics and Confucianism. *Comparative Approaches to Chinese Philosophy* 2003;23:99–121.

6. Stiefel F, Bourquin C. Moving toward the next generation of communication training in oncology: The relevance of findings from qualitative research. *Eur J Cancer Care (Engl)* 2019;28(6):e13149. https://doi.org/10.1111/ecc.13149.

7. Gulbrandsen P, Gerwing J, Landmark AM. Time to advance the educational model of clinical communication in medicine. *Patient Educ Couns* 2022;105(6):1351–2.

8. Kinghorn WA. Medical education as moral formation: An Aristotelian account of medical professionalsim. *Perspect Biol Med* 2010;53(1):87–105.

9. Kotzee B, Paton A, Conroy M. Towards an empirically informed account of phronesis in medicine. *Perspect Biol Med* 2016;59(3):337–50.

10. Kleinman A. Moral experience and ethical reflection: Can ethnography reconcile them? A quandary for 'the new bioethics'. *Daedalus* 1999;128(4):69–97.

11. Giorgetti A. Between the Doctor and the Patient: History of the Relationship. In Pingitore A, Iacono AM, eds. *The Patient as a Person: An Integrated and Systemic Approach to Patient and Disease.* Cham: Springer 2023: 3–13.

12. Kleinman A. *The Illness Narratives: Suffering, Healing, and the Human Condition.* New York: Basic Books 2020.

13. Pilnick A. Reconsidering patient-centred care: Authority, expertise and abandonment. *Health Expect* 2023;26(5):1785–8. https://doi.org/10.1111/hex.13815.

14. Katz J. *The Silent World of Doctor and Patient.* New York: The Free Press 1984.

15. Murray PM. The history of informed consent. *Iowa Orthopedic J* 1990;10:104–9.

16. Dunn M, Fulford KWM, Herring J, et al. Between the reasonable and the particular: Deflating autonomy in the legal regulation of informed consent to medical treatment. *Health Care Anal* 2019;27(2):110–27. https://doi.org/10.1007/s10728-018-0358-x.

17. Botti C, Vaccari A. End-of-life decision-making and advance care directives in Italy. A report and moral appraisal of recent legal provisions. *Bioethics* 27:110–27 https://doi.org/10.1111/bioe.12615.

18. Turillazzi E, Neri M, Riezzo I, et al. Informed Consent in Italy-Traditional Versus the Law: A Gordian Knot. *Aesthetic Plast Surg* 2014;38(4):759–64. https://doi.org/10.1007/s00266-014-0337-z.

19. Bozzola E, Spina G, Russo R, et al. Mandatory vaccinations in European countries, undocumented information, false news and the impact on vaccination uptake: The position of the Italian pediatric society. *Ital J Pediatr* 2018;44(1):67. https://doi.org/10.1186/s13052-018-0504-y.

20. Gibelli F, Ricci G, Sirignano A, et al. COVID-19 compulsory vaccination: Legal and bioethical controversies. *Front Med (Lausanne)* 2022;9:821522. https://doi.org/10.3389/fmed.2022.821522.

21. Chirico F. The new Italian mandatory vaccine Law as a health policy instrument against the anti-vaccination movement. *Ann Ig* 2018;30(3):251–6. https://doi.org/10.7416/ai.2018.2217.

22. Williams BM. The ethics of selective mandatory vaccination for COVID-19. *Public Health Ethics* 2022;15(1):74–86. https://doi.org/10.1093/phe/phab028.

23. Beauchamp TL, Childress JF. *Principles of Biomedical Ethics.* Oxford: Oxford University Press 1979.

24. Goldstein MM, Bowers DG. The patient as consumer: Empowerment or commodification? *J Law Med Ethics* 2015;43(1):162–5. https://doi.org/10.1111/jlme.12203.

25. Martinez MJ, Dixit D, White MW, et al. Motivations for seeking cosmetic enhancing procedures of the face: A systematic review. *Dermatol Surg* 2023;49(3):278–82. https://doi.org/10.1097/dss.0000000000003702.

26. Locatelli K, Boccara D, De Runz A, et al. A qualitative study of life events and psychological needs underlying the decision to have cosmetic surgery. *Int J Psychiatry Med* 2017;52(1):88–105. https://doi.org/10.1177/0091217417703287.

27. Gilbar R, Miola J. One size fits all? On patient autonomy, medical decision-making, and the impact of culture. *Med Law Rev* 2015;23 (3):375–99.

28. Degner LF, Sloan JA. Decision making during serious illness: What role do patients really want to play? *J Clin Epidemiol* 1992;45(9):941–50.

29. Meredith C, Symonds P, Webster L, et al. Information needs of cancer patients in west Scotland: cross sectional survey of patients' views. *Br Med J* 1996;313(7059):724–6. https://doi.org/10.1136/bmj.313.7059.724.

30. Rankin N, Newell S, Sanson-Fisher R, et al. Consumer participation in the development of psychosocial clinical practice guidelines: Opinions of women with breast cancer. *Eur J Cancer Care (Engl)* 2000;9(2):97–104.

31. Rosenbaum L. The paternalism preference – Choosing unshared decision making. *N Engl J Med* 2015;373(7):589–92. https://doi.org/10.1056/ NEJMp1508418.

32. Salander P, Henriksson R. Severely diseased lung cancer patients narrate the importance of being included in a helping relationship. *Lung Cancer* 2005;50(2):155–62.

33. Skelton JR. *Language and Clinical Communication: This Bright Babylon*. Abingdon: Radcliffe 2008.

34. Paul KT, Zimmermann BM, Corsico P, et al. Anticipating hopes, fears and expectations towards COVID-19 vaccines: A qualitative interview study in seven European countries. *SSM Qual Res Health* 2022;2:100035. https:// doi.org/10.1016/j.ssmqr.2021.100035.

35. Carter SM, Entwistle VA, Little M. Relational conceptions of paternalism: a way to rebut nanny-state accusations and evaluate public health interventions. *Public Health* 2015;129(8):1021–9. https://doi.org/ 10.1016/j.puhe.2015.03.007.

36. Entwistle VA, Carter SM, Cribb A, et al. Supporting Patient Autonomy: The importance of clinician-patient relationships. *J Gen Intern Med* 2010;25(7):741–5. https://doi.org/10.1007/s11606-010-1292-2.

37. Entwistle VA, Prior M, Skea ZC, et al. Involvement in treatment decision-making: Its meaning to people with diabetes and implications for conceptualisation. *Soc Sci Med* 2008;66(2):362–75. https://doi.org/ S0277-9536(07)00500-X [pii]10.1016/j.socscimed.2007.09.001.

38. Dove ES, Kelly SE, Lucivero F, et al. Beyond individualism: Is there a place for relational autonomy in clinical practice and research? *Clin Ethics* 2017;12(3):150–65.

39. Orfali K, Gordon EJ. Autonomy gone awry: a cross-cultural study of parents' experiences in neonatal intensive care units. *Theor Med Bioeth* 2004;25(4):329–65. https://doi.org/10.1007/s11017-004-3135-9.

40. Kukla R. Conscientious autonomy – Displacing decisions in health care. *Hastings Cent Rep* 2005;35(2):34–44.

41. Mendick N, Young B, Holcombe C, et al. The ethics of responsibility and ownership in decision-making about treatment for breast cancer: Triangulation of consultation with patient and surgeon perspectives. *Soc Sci Med* 2010;70(12):1904–11. https://doi.org/S0277-9536(10)00225-X [pii]10.1016/j.socscimed.2009.12.039.

42. Beach MC, Branyon E, Saha S. Diverse patient perspectives on respect in healthcare: A qualitative study. *Patient Educ Couns* 2017;100(11):2076–80. https://doi.org/10.1016/j.pec.2017.05.010.

43. Entwistle VA, Cribb A, Mitchell P. Tackling disrespect in health care: The relevance of socio-relational equality. *J Health Serv Res Policy* 2024;29 (1):42–50. https://doi.org/10.1177/13558196231187961.

44. Beach MC, Duggan PS, Cassel CK, et al. What does 'respect' mean? Exploring the moral obligation of health professionals to respect patients. *J Gen Intern Med* 2007;22(5):692–5. https://doi.org/10.1007/s11606-006-0054-7.

45. Pellegrino ED. The virtuous physician, and the ethics of medicine. In Shelp EE, ed. *Virtue and medicine. Philosophy and Medicine.* Dordrecht: Springer 1985:237–55.

46. Turoldo F. Relational autonomy and multiculturalism. *Camb Q Healthc Ethics* 2010;19(4):542–9. https://doi.org/10.1017/S0963180110000496.

47. Nakata Y, Goto T, Morita S. Serving the emperor without asking: Critical care ethics in Japan. *J Med Philos* 1998;23(6):601–15. https://doi.org/10.1076/jmep.23.6.601.2557.

48. Engel GL. The need for a new medical model: A challenge for biomedicine. *Science* 1977;196(4286):129–36. https://doi.org/10.1126/science.847460.

49. Salmon P, Young B. Dependence and caring in clinical communication: The relevance of attachment and other theories. *Patient Educ Couns* 2009;74(3):331–8. https://doi.org/S0738-3991(08)00650-2 [pii]10.1016/j .pec.2008.12.011.

50. Stiefel F, Barth J, Bensing J, et al. Communication skills training in oncology: a position paper based on a consensus meeting among European experts in 2009. *Ann Oncol* 2010;21(2):204–7. https://doi.org/ mdp564[pii]10.1093/annonc/mdp564.

51. Levinson W, Gorawara-Bhat R, Lamb J. A study of patient clues and physician responses in primary care and surgical settings. *JAMA* 2000;284(8):1021–7.

52. Hsu I, Saha S, Korthuis PT, et al. Providing support to patients in emotional encounters: A new perspective on missed empathic opportunities. *Patient Educ Couns* 2012;88(3):436–42.

53. Kuchinad K, Park JR, Han D, et al. Which clinician responses to emotion are associated with more positive patient experiences of communication? *Patient Educ Couns* 2024:108241.

54. Stepien KA, Baernstein A. Educating for empathy. *J Gen Intern Med* 2006;21(5):524–30. https://doi.org/10.1111/j.1525-1497.2006.00443.x.

55. Stiefel F. Support of the supporters. *Support Care Cancer* 2008;16(2):123–6. https://doi.org/10.1007/s00520-007-0355-3.

56. Stiefel F, Bourquin C, Salmon P, et al. Communication and support of patients and caregivers in chronic cancer care: ESMO Clinical Practice Guideline☆. *ESMO Open* 2024;9(7):103496. https://doi.org/10.1016/j.esmoop.2024.103496.

57. Young B, Ward J, Forsey M, et al. Examining the validity of the unitary theory of clinical relationships: comparison of observed and experienced parent-doctor interaction. *Patient Educ Couns* 2011;85(1):60–7. https://doi.org/S0738-3991(10)00548-3 [pii]10.1016/j.pec.2010.08.027.

58. Brandes K, van der Goot MJ, Smit EG, et al. Understanding the interplay of cancer patients' instrumental concerns and emotions. *Patient Educ Couns* 2017;100(5):839–45.

59. Semmer NK, Elfering A, Jacobshagen N, et al. The emotional meaning of instrumental social support. *Int J Stress Management* 2008;15(3):235–51.

60. Salmon P, Humphris GM, Ring A, et al. Why do primary care physicians propose medical care to patients with medically unexplained symptoms? A new method of sequence analysis to test theories of patient pressure. *Psychosom Med* 2006;68(4):570–7.

61. Salvadé H, Stiefel F, Bourquin C. 'You'll need to settle your affairs': How the subject of death is approached by oncologists and advanced cancer patients in follow-up consultations. *Pall Support Care* 2022;22:655–63. https://doi.org/10.1017/S147895152200147X.

62. McWilliam CL, Brown JB, Stewart M. Breast cancer patients' experiences of patient-doctor communication: a working relationship. *Patient Educ Couns* 2000;39(2–3):191–204.

63. Palmer Kelly E, Tsilimigras DI, Hyer JM, et al. Understanding the use of attachment theory applied to the patient-provider relationship in cancer care: Recommendations for future research and clinical practice. *Surg Oncol* 2019;31:101–10. https://doi.org/10.1016/j.suronc.2019.10.007.

64. Tan A, Zimmermann C, Rodin G. Interpersonal processes in palliative care: An attachment perspective on the patient-clinician relationship. *Palliat Med* 2005;19(2):143–50.

65. Maunder RG, Hunter JJ. Can patients be 'attached' to healthcare providers? An observational study to measure attachment phenomena in patient-provider relationships. *BMJ Open* 2016;6(5):e011068. https://doi.org/10.1136/bmjopen-2016-011068.

66. Bowlby J. *Attachment and Loss Vol 1. Attachment.* 2nd ed. New York: Basic Books 1982.

67. Bowlby J. *A Secure Base: Clinical Applications of Attachment Theory.* London: Routledge 1988.

68. Mikulincer M, Shaver PR. *Attachment in Adulthood: Structure, Dynamics, and Change.* 2nd ed. New York: Guilford Press 2016.

69. Mikulincer M, Shaver PR. The attachment behavioral system in adulthood: Activation, psychodynamics, and interpersonal processes. *Adv Exp Soc Psychol* 2003;35:53–152.

70. Birtchnell J. Attachment in an interpersonal context. *Br J Med Psychol* 1997;70 (Pt 3):265–79; discussion 81–90.

71. Young B, Hill J, Gravenhorst K, et al. Is communication guidance mistaken? Qualitative study of parent-oncologist communication in childhood cancer. *Br J Cancer* 2013;109(4):836–43. https://doi.org/10.1038/bjc.2013.413.

72. Salmon P, Young B. The inseparability of emotional and instrumental care in cancer: Towards a more powerful science of clinical communication. *Patient Educ Couns* 2017;100(11):2138–40. https://doi.org/10.1016/j.pec.2017.05.019.

73. Wright EB, Holcombe C, Salmon P. Doctors communication of trust, care, and respect in breast cancer: qualitative study. *Br Med J* 2004;328 (7444):864–7.

74. Milberg A, Wahlberg R, Jakobsson M, et al. What is a 'secure base' when death is approaching? A study applying attachment theory to adult patients' and family members' experiences of palliative home care. *Psychooncology* 2012;21(8):886–95. https://doi.org/10.1002/pon.1982.

75. Ricco B, Fiorani C, Ferrara L, et al. Survey on the effectiveness of telephone-based communication with relatives of hospitalized cancer patients in COVID-19 era in Italy. *Support Care Cancer* 2022;30 (7):6007–12. https://doi.org/10.1007/s00520-022-07042-1.

76. Borghi L. Clinician-patient-family member interactions in COVID-19 serious conditions: A glimpse from the other side of the limbo. *Patient Educ Couns* 2021;104(8):1887–8. https://doi.org/10.1016/j.pec.2021.02.003.

77. Griffin D, Bartholomew K. Models of the self and other – Fundamental dimensions underlying measures of adult attachment. *J Pers Soc Psychol* 1994;67(3):430–45.

78. Ciechanowski PS, Walker EA, Katon WJ, et al. Attachment theory: A model for health care utilization and somatization. *Psychosom Med* 2002;64(4):660–7.

79. Ciechanowski PS, Worley LL, Russo JE, et al. Using relationship styles based on attachment theory to improve understanding of specialty choice in medicine. *BMC Med Educ* 2006;6:3.

80. Bartholomew K, Horowitz LM. Attachment styles among young adults: A test of a four-category model. *J Pers Soc Psychol* 1991;61(2):226–44.

81. Ciechanowski P, Katon WJ. The interpersonal experience of health care through the eyes of patients with diabetes. *Soc Sci Med* 2006;63(12):3067–79. https://doi.org/S0277-9536(06)00404-7 [pii]10.1016/j.socscimed.2006.08.002.

82. Ciechanowski PS. As fundamental as nouns and verbs? Towards an integration of attachment theory in medical training. *Med Educ* 2010;44(2):122–4.

83. Ciechanowski P, Katon WJ. The interpersonal experience of health care through the eyes of patients with diabetes. *Soc Sci Med* 2006;63(12):3067–79. https://doi.org/10.1016/j.socscimed.2006.08.002.

84. Hunter J, Maunder R. *Improving Patient Treatment with Attachment Theory: A Guide for Primary Care Practitioners and Specialists*. Switzerland: Springer 2015.

85. Zaporowska-Stachowiak I, Stachowiak K, Stachnik K. Two is a perfect number: Patient–doctor relationship and patient attachment style in palliative care. *J Health Psychol* 2019;24(5):549–60. https://doi.org/10.1177/1359105317721307.

86. Forsey M, Salmon P, Eden T, et al. Comparing doctors' and nurses' accounts of how they provide emotional care for parents of children with acute lymphoblastic leukaemia. *Psychooncology* 2013;22(2):260–7. https://doi.org/10.1002/pon.2084.

87. Fletcher I, McCallum R, Peters S. Attachment styles and clinical communication performance in trainee doctors. *Patient Educ Couns* 2016;99(11):1852–7. https://doi.org/10.1016/j.pec.2016.05.019.

88. Ciechanowski PS, Russo JE, Katon WJ, et al. Attachment theory in health care: The influence of relationship style on medical students' specialty choice. *Med Educ* 2004;38(3):262–70.

89. Salmon P, Wissow L, Carroll J, et al. Doctors' responses to patients with medically unexplained symptoms who seek emotional support: criticism or confrontation? *Gen Hosp Psychiatry* 2007;29(5):454–60.

90. Salmon P, Wissow L, Carroll J, et al. Doctors' attachment style and their inclination to propose somatic interventions for medically unexplained symptoms. *Gen Hosp Psychiatry* 2008;30(2):104–11.

91. Cherry MG, Fletcher I, O'Sullivan H. The influence of medical students' and doctors' attachment style and emotional intelligence on their patient–provider communication. *Patient Educ Couns* 2013;93(2):177–87. https://doi.org/10.1016/j.pec.2013.05.010.

92. Cherry MG, Fletcher I, Berridge D, et al. Do doctors' attachment styles and emotional intelligence influence patients' emotional expressions in primary care consultations? An exploratory study using multilevel analysis. *Patient Educ Couns* 2018;101(4):659–64. https://doi.org/10.1016/j.pec.2017.10.017.

93. Adshead G. Becoming a caregiver: Attachment theory and poorly performing doctors. *Med Educ* 2010;44(2):125–31. https://doi.org/10.1111/j.1365-2923.2009.03556.x.

94. Granek L, Shapira S, Constantini S, et al. 'Every patient is like my child': Pediatric neurosurgeons' relational and emotional bonds with their patients and families. *Br J Neurosurg* 2022;36(1):70–4. https://doi.org/10.1080/02688697.2021.1958156.

95. Terrasson J, Seigneur E, Rault A, et al. The announcement of treatment resistance from the pediatric oncologist's point of view: A qualitative study. *Pediatr Hematol Oncol* 2022;39(2):132–44. https://doi.org/10.1080/08880018.2021.1956030.

96. Kelly BJ, Varghese FT, Pelusi D. Countertransference and ethics: A perspective on clinical dilemmas in end-of-life decisions. *Palliat Support Care* 2003;1(4):367–75.

97. Balint M. The doctor, his patient and the illness. London: Pitman Medical 1957.

98. Balint M. The doctor's therapeutic function. *Lancet* 1965;1(7397):1177–80.

99. Sally AH. Balint work and the flourishing practitioner. *Br J Gen Pract* 2023;73(732):323. https://doi.org/10.3399/bjgp23X733449.

100. Van Roy K, Vanheule S, Inslegers R. Research on Balint groups: A literature review. *Patient Educ Couns* 2015;98(6):685–94. https://doi.org/10.1016/j.pec.2015.01.014.

101. Passalacqua R, Campione F, Caminiti C, et al. Patients' opinions, feelings, and attitudes after a campaign to promote the Di Bella therapy. *Lancet* 1999;353(9161):1310–4. https://doi.org/10.1016/S0140-6736(98)10253-2.

102. Soothill K, Wilson D. Theorising the puzzle that is Harold Shipman. *J Forensic Psychiatr Psychol* 2005;16(4):685–98. https://doi.org/10.1080/14789940500282467.

103. Fumagalli LP, Radaelli G, Lettieri E, et al. Patient Empowerment and its neighbours: Clarifying the boundaries and their mutual relationships. *Health Pol* 2015;119(3):384–94. https://doi.org/10.1016/j.healthpol.2014.10.017.

104. Pekonen A, Eloranta S, Stolt M, et al. Measuring patient empowerment – A systematic review. *Patient Educ Couns* 2020;103(4):777–87. https://doi.org/10.1016/j.pec.2019.10.019.

105. Hickmann E, Richter P, Schlieter H. All together now–patient engagement, patient empowerment, and associated terms in personal healthcare. *BMC Health Serv Res* 2022;22(1):1116.

106. Pekonen A, Eloranta S, Stolt M, et al. Measuring patient empowerment–A systematic review. *Patient Educ Couns* 2020;103(4):777–87.

107. Kinney RL, Lemon SC, Person SD, et al. The association between patient activation and medication adherence, hospitalization, and emergency room utilization in patients with chronic illnesses: a systematic review. *Patient Educ Couns* 2015;98(5):545–52. https://doi.org/10.1016/j.pec.2015.02.005.

108. Barnes EL, Long MD, Kappelman MD, et al. High patient activation is associated with remission in patients with inflammatory bowel disease. *Inflamm Bowel Dis* 2019;25(7):1248–54. https://doi.org/10.1093/ibd/izy378.

109. Hibbard JH, Greene J, Shi Y, et al. Taking the long view: How well do patient activation scores predict outcomes four years later? *Med Care Res Rev* 2015;72(3):324–37. https://doi.org/10.1177/1077558715573871.

110. Greene J, Hibbard JH. Why does patient activation matter? An examination of the relationships between patient activation and health-related outcomes. *J Gen Intern Med* 2012;27(5):520–6. https://doi.org/10.1007/s11606-011-1931-2.

111. Ng APP, Cheng JKY, Lam JSM, et al. Patient enablement and health-related quality of life for patients with chronic back and knee pain: A cross-sectional study in primary care. *Br J Gen Pract* 2023;73(736):e867–e75. https://doi.org/10.3399/bjgp.2022.0546.

112. Ernstmann N, Wirtz M, Nitzsche A, et al. Patients' trust in physician, patient enablement, and health-related quality of life during colon cancer treatment. *J Cancer Educ* 2017;32(3):571–9. https://doi.org/10.1007/s13187-017-1166-y.

113. Mercer SW, Neumann M, Wirtz M, et al. General practitioner empathy, patient enablement, and patient-reported outcomes in primary care in an area of high socio-economic deprivation in Scotland—A pilot prospective study using structural equation modeling. *Patient Educ Couns* 2008;73(2):240–5. https://doi.org/10.1016/j.pec.2008.07.022.

114. Tolvanen E, Koskela TH, Kosunen E. Comparison of the Patient Enablement Instrument (PEI) with two single-item measures among

Finnish Health care centre patients. *BMC Health Serv Res* 2019;19 (1):376. https://doi.org/10.1186/s12913-019-4182-2.

115. Hibbard JH, Stockard J, Mahoney ER, et al. Development of the Patient Activation Measure (PAM): Conceptualizing and measuring activation in patients and consumers. *Health Serv Res* 2004;39(4p1):1005–26. https://doi.org/10.1111/j.1475-6773.2004.00269.x.

116. Lin MY, Weng WS, Apriliyasari RW, et al. Effects of patient activation intervention on chronic diseases: A meta-analysis. *J Nurs Res* 2020;28(5): e116. https://doi.org/10.1097/jnr.0000000000000387.

117. Lorig K, Ritter PL, Turner RM, et al. A Diabetes self-management program: 12-month outcome sustainability from a nonreinforced pragmatic trial. *J Med Internet Res* 2016;18(12):e322. https://doi.org/10.2196/jmir.6484.

118. Bodenheimer T, Wagner EH, Grumbach K. Improving primary care for patients with chronic illness. *JAMA* 2002;288(14):1775–9. https://doi.org/10.1001/jama.288.14.1775.

119. Petrelli F, Cangelosi G, Nittari G, et al. Chronic care model in Italy: A narrative review of the literature. *Prim Health Care Res Dev* 2021;22: e32. https://doi.org/10.1017/S1463423621000268.

120. Lorig K, Ritter PL, Laurent DD, et al. Online diabetes self-management program: A randomized study. *Diabetes Care* 2010;33(6):1275–81. https://doi.org/10.2337/dc09-2153.

121. Regeer H, van Empelen P, Bilo HJ, et al. Change is possible: How increased patient activation is associated with favorable changes in well-being, self-management and health outcomes among people with type 2 diabetes mellitus: A prospective longitudinal study. *Patient Educ Couns* 2022;105 (4):821–7.

122. Frost J, Currie MJ, Cruickshank M. An integrative review of enablement in primary health care. *J Prim Care Community Health* 2015;6(4):264–78. https://doi.org/10.1177/2150131915598373.

123. Lindsay A, Hibbard JH, Boothroyd DB, et al. Patient activation changes as a potential signal for changes in health care costs: Cohort study of US high-cost patients. *J Gen Intern Med* 2018;33(12):2106–12. https://doi.org/10.1007/s11606-018-4657-6.

124. Salmon P, Hall GM. Patient empowerment and control: A psychological discourse in the service of medicine. *Soc Sci Med* 2003;57(10):1969–80.

125. Sinding C, Hudak P, Wiernikowski J, et al. 'I like to be an informed person but . . . ' negotiating responsibility for treatment decisions in cancer care. *Soc Sci Med* 2010;71(6):1094–101. https://doi.org/10.1016/j.socscimed.2010 .06.005.

126. Axon A. Ethical considerations in gastroenterology and endoscopy. *Dig Dis* 2003;20(3–4):220–5. https://doi.org/10.1159/000067671.
127. Reid J. *Choice for All, Not the Few.* London: Department of Health, 2003.
128. Newland P, Lorenz R, Oliver BJ. Patient activation in adults with chronic conditions: A systematic review. *J Health Psychol* 2021;26(1):103–14. https://doi.org/10.1177/1359105320947790.
129. Charles C, Gafni A, Whelan T. Shared decision-making in the medical encounter: What does it mean? (or it takes at least two to tango). *Soc Sci Med* 1997;44(5):681–92. https://doi.org/S0277953696002213 [pii].
130. Charles C, Gafni A, Whelan T. Decision-making in the physician-patient encounter: Revisiting the shared treatment decision-making model. *Soc Sci Med* 1999;49(5):651–61. https://doi.org/S0277953699001458[pii].
131. Elwyn G, Frosch D, Thomson R, et al. Shared decision making: A model for clinical practice. *J Gen Intern Med* 2012;27(10):1361–7. https://doi.org/10.1007/s11606-012-2077-6.
132. Elwyn G, Miron-Shatz T. Deliberation before determination: The definition and evaluation of good decision making. *Health Expect* 2010;13(2):139–47. https://doi.org/10.1111/j.1369-7625.2009.00572.x.
133. Elwyn G, Lloyd A, May C, et al. Collaborative deliberation: A model for patient care. *Patient Educ Couns* 2014;97(2):158–64. https://doi.org/10.1016/j.pec.2014.07.027.
134. Couët N, Desroches S, Robitaille H, et al. Assessments of the extent to which health-care providers involve patients in decision making: A systematic review of studies using the OPTION instrument. *Health Expect* 2015;18(4):542–61. https://doi.org/10.1111/hex.12054.
135. Gerwing J, Gulbrandsen P. Contextualizing decisions: Stepping out of the SDM track. *Patient Educ Couns* 2019;102(5):815–16. https://doi.org/10.1016/j.pec.2019.03.024.
136. Beach MC, Sugarman J. Realizing shared decision-making in practice. *JAMA* 2019;322(9):811. https://doi.org/10.1001/jama.2019.9797.
137. Brown SL, Salmon P. Reconciling the theory and reality of shared decision-making: A "matching" approach to practitioner leadership. *Health Expect* 2019;22(3):275–83. https://doi.org/10.1111/hex.12853.
138. Entwistle VA, Watt IS. Patient involvement in treatment decision-making: The case for a broader conceptual framework. *Patient Educ Couns* 2006;63(3):268–78. https://doi.org/S0738-3991(06)00156-X [pii]10.1016/j.pec.2006.05.002.
139. Landry JT. Current models of shared decision-making are insufficient: The 'Professionally-Driven Zone of Patient or Surrogate Discretion'

offers a defensible way forward. *Patient Educ Couns* 2023;115:107892. https://doi.org/10.1016/j.pec.2023.107892.

140. Graff V, Clapp JT, Heins SJ, et al. Patient Involvement in Anesthesia Decision-making: A qualitative study of knee arthroplasty. *Anesthesiol* 2021;135(1):111–21. https://doi.org/10.1097/ALN.0000000000003795.

141. Thomas EC, Bass SB, Siminoff LA. Beyond rationality: Expanding the practice of shared decision making in modern medicine. *Soc Sci Med* 2021;277:113900.

142. Eirik Hugaas O, Jan CF, Edvin S, et al. Clinical decisions presented to patients in hospital encounters: A cross-sectional study using a novel taxonomy. *BMJ Open* 2018;8(1):e018042. https://doi.org/10.1136/bmjo pen-2017-018042.

143. Peerbhoy D, Hall GM, Parker C, et al. Patients' reactions to attempts to increase passive or active coping with surgery. *Soc Sci Med* 1998;47 (5):595–601.

144. Gigerenzer G, Gaissmaier W. Heuristic decision making. *Ann Rev Psychol* 2011;62(1):451–82. https://doi.org/10.1146/annurev-psych-120709-145346.

145. Keshtgar A, Cunningham SJ, Jones E, et al. Patient, clinician and independent observer perspectives of shared decision making in adult orthodontics. *J Orthod* 2021;48(4):417–25. https://doi.org/10.1177/14653125211007504.

146. Scholl I, Kriston L, Dirmaier J, et al. Comparing the nine-item shared decision-making questionnaire to the OPTION scale –An attempt to establish convergent validity. *Health Expect* 2015;18(1):137–50. https://doi.org/10.1111/hex.12022.

147. Saba GW, Wong ST, Schillinger D, et al. Shared decision making and the experience of partnership in primary care. *Ann Fam Med* 2006;4(1):54–62. https://doi.org/10.1370/afm.393.

148. Légaré F, Adekpedjou R, Stacey D, et al. Interventions for increasing the use of shared decision making by healthcare professionals. *Cochrane Database Syst Rev* 2018(7):CD006732. https://doi.org/10.1002/14651858.CD006732.pub4.

149. Shay LA, Lafata JE. Where is the evidence? A systematic review of shared decision making and patient outcomes. *Med Decis Making* 2015;35(1):114–31.

150. Mathijssen EG, van den Bemt BJ, van den Hoogen FH, et al. Interventions to support shared decision making for medication therapy in long term conditions: A systematic review. *Patient Educ Couns* 2020;103(2):254–65.

151. Vaseur RM, Te Braake E, Beinema T, et al. Technology-supported shared decision-making in chronic conditions: A systematic review of randomized controlled trials. *Patient Educ Couns* 2024;124:108267.

152. Bruch JD, Khazen M, Mahmic-Kaknjo M, et al. The effects of shared decision making on health outcomes, health care quality, cost, and consultation time: An umbrella review. *Patient Educ Couns* 2024;129:108408. https://doi.org/10.1016/j.pec.2024.108408.

153. Elwyn G, Frosch D, Volandes AE, et al. Investing in deliberation: A definition and classification of decision support interventions for people facing difficult health decisions. *Med Decis Making* 2010;30(6):701–11.

154. Leinweber KA, Columbo JA, Kang R, et al. A review of decision aids for patients considering more than one type of invasive treatment. *J Surg Res* 2019;235:350–66. https://doi.org/10.1016/j.jss.2018.09.017.

155. Stacey D, Lewis KB, Smith M, et al. Decision aids for people facing health treatment or screening decisions. *Cochrane Database Syst Rev* 2017;4(4): CD001431. https://doi.org/10.1002/14651858.CD001431 .pub5.

156. Gans EA, van Mun LA, de Groot JF, et al. Supporting older patients in making healthcare decisions: The effectiveness of decision aids; A systematic review and meta-analysis. *Patient Educ Couns* 2023;116:107981.

157. Eltorai AEM, Naqvi SS, Ghanian S, et al. Readability of invasive procedure consent forms. *Clin Transl Sci* 2015;8(6):830–3. https://doi.org/ 10.1111/cts.12364.

158. Duong Q, Mandrekar SJ, Winham SJ, et al. Understanding verbosity: Funding source and the length of consent forms for cancer clinical trials. *J Cancer Educ* 2021;36(6):1248–52. https://doi.org/10.1007/s13187-020-01757-7.

159. Matlock DD, Fukunaga MI, Tan A, et al. Enhancing success of Medicare's shared decision making mandates using implementation science: Examples applying the pragmatic robust implementation and sustainability model (PRISM). *MDM Policy & Practice* 2020;5(2):2381468320963070. https://doi.org/10.1177/2381468320963070.

160. Joseph-Williams N, Elwyn G, Edwards A. Knowledge is not power for patients: A systematic review and thematic synthesis of patient-reported barriers and facilitators to shared decision making. *Patient Educ Couns* 2014;94(3):291–309. https://doi.org/10.1016/j.pec.2013.10.031.

161. Entwistle VA, Carter SM, Trevena L, et al. Communicating about screening. *Br Med J* 2008;337:a1591.

162. Galasiński D, Ziółkowska J, Elwyn G. Epistemic justice is the basis of shared decision making. *Patient Educ Couns* 2023;111:107681.

163. Pieterse AH, Gulbrandsen P, Ofstad EH, et al. What does shared decision making ask from doctors? Uncovering suppressed qualities that could improve person-centered care. *Patient Educ Couns* 2023; 114:107801.

164. Levenstein JH, McCracken EC, McWhinney IR, et al. The patient-centred clinical method. 1. A model for the doctor-patient interaction in family medicine. *Fam Pract* 1986;3(1):24–30. https://doi.org/10.1093/fampra/ 3.1.24.

165. Brown J, Stewart M, McCracken E, et al. The patient-centred clinical method. 2. definition and application. *Fam Pract* 1986;3(2):75–9. https:// doi.org/10.1093/fampra/3.2.75.

166. Stewart M, Brown JB, Weston WW. Patient-centred interviewing part III: Five provocative questions. *Can Fam Physician* 1989;35:159–61.

167. Mead N, Bower P. Patient-centredness: A conceptual framework and review of the empirical literature. *Soc Sci Med* 2000;51(7):1087–110. http://dx.doi.org/10.1016/S0277-9536(00)00098-8.

168. The Health Foundation. *Person-Centred Care Made Simple: What Everyone should know about Person-Centred Care.* London: The Health Foundation 2015.

169. Dwamena F, Holmes-Rovner M, Gaulden CM, et al. Interventions for providers to promote a patient-centred approach in clinical consultations. *Cochrane Database Syst Rev* 2012(12). https://doi.org/10.1002/ 14651858.CD003267.pub2.

170. Chew-Graham CA, May CR, Roland MO. The harmful consequences of elevating the doctor-patient relationship to be a primary goal of the general practice consultation. *Fam Pract* 2004;21(3):229–31.

171. Miller BM, Fritz Z. In this uncertain world, patient-centred care must not mean patient-led care. *Br J Gen Pract* 2019;69(682):259–60. https://doi.org/ 10.3399/bjgp19X702641.

172. Bansal A, Greenley S, Mitchell C, et al. Optimising planned medical education strategies to develop learners' Person-Centredness: A realist review. *Med Educ* 2022;56(5):489–503.

173. Makoul G, Noble L, Gulbrandsen P, et al. Reinforcing the humanity in healthcare: The Glasgow Consensus Statement on effective communication in clinical encounters. *Patient Educ Couns* 2024;122:108158. https:// doi.org/10.1016/j.pec.2024.108158.

174. Argyle M, ed. *Social Skills and Health.* London: Methuen 1981.

175. Argyle M. *The Psychology of Interpersonal Behaviour.* Harmondsworth: Penguin 1967.

176. Langewitz W. Beyond content analysis and non-verbal behaviour. What about atmosphere?: A phenomenological approach. *Patient Educ Couns* 2007;67(3):319–23.

177. Makoul G. Communication skills education in medical school and beyond. *JAMA* 2003;289(1):93. https://doi.org/10.1001/jama.289.1.93.

178. Brown J. How clinical communication has become a core part of medical education in the UK. *Med Educ* 2008;42(3):271–8. https://doi.org/10.1111/j.1365-2923.2007.02955.x.

179. Simpson M, Buckman R, Stewart M, et al. Doctor-patient communication – The Toronto consensus statement. *Br Med J* 1991;303(6814):1385–7.

180. Maguire P. Improving communication with cancer patients. *Eur J Cancer* 1999;35(10):1415–22. https://doi.org/10.1016/s0959-8049(99)00178-1.

181. Fallowfield L, Jenkins V. Effective communication skills are the key to good cancer care. *Eur J Cancer* 1999;35(11):1592–7.

182. Baile WF, Aaron J. Patient-physician communication in oncology: Past, present, and future. *Curr Opin Oncol* 2005;17(4):331–5. https://doi.org/10.1097/01.cco.0000167738.49325.2c.

183. Bylund CL, Brown R, Gueguen JA, et al. The implementation and assessment of a comprehensive communication skills training curriculum for oncologists. *Psychooncology* 2010;19(6):583–93. https://doi.org/10.1002/pon.1585.

184. von Fragstein M, Silverman J, Cushing A, et al. UK consensus statement on the content of communication curricula in undergraduate medical education. *Med Educ* 2008;42(11):1100–7. https://doi.org/10.1111/j.1365-2923.2008.03137.x.

185. Bachmann C, Abramovitch H, Barbu CG, et al. A European consensus on learning objectives for a core communication curriculum in health care professions. *Patient Educ Couns* 2013;93(1):18–26. https://doi.org/10.1016/j.pec.2012.10.016.

186. Street RL, De Haes H. Designing a curriculum for communication skills training from a theory and evidence-based perspective. *Patient Educ Couns* 2013;93(1):27–33. https://doi.org/10.1016/j.pec.2013.06.012.

187. Kurtz S, Silverman J, Benson J, et al. Marrying content and process in clinical method teaching: enhancing the Calgary-Cambridge guides. *Acad Med* 2003;78(8):802–9. https://doi.org/10.1097/00001888-200308000-00011.

188. Yuen JK, See C, Cheung JTK, et al. Can teaching serious illness communication skills foster multidimensional empathy? A mixed-methods study. *BMC Med Educ* 2023;23(1):20. https://doi.org/10.1186/s12909-023-04010-z.

189. van Weel-Baumgarten EM, Brouwers M, Grosfeld F, et al. Teaching and training in breaking bad news at the Dutch medical schools: A comparison. *Med Teach* 2012;34(5):373–81. https://doi.org/10.3109/0142159X.2012.668247.

190. Aurora O, Susan EM. Training programs for improving communication about medical research and clinical trials: A systematic review. In Milica P, ed. *Clinical Trials in Vulnerable Populations*. Rijeka: IntechOpen 2017:Ch. 11.

191. Stiefel F, Bourquin C. Communication in oncology: Now we train – but how well? *Ann Oncol* 2016;27(9):1660–3. https://doi.org/10.1093/annonc/mdw229.

192. Stiefel F, Kiss A, Salmon P, et al. Training in communication of oncology clinicians: a position paper based on the third consensus meeting among European experts in 2018. *Ann Oncol* 2018;29(10):2033–6. https://doi.org/10.1093/annonc/mdy343.

193. Bales RF. A set of categories for the analysis of small group interaction. *Am Sociol Rev* 1950;15(2):257. https://doi.org/10.2307/2086790.

194. Bales RF. *Interaction Process Analysis: A Method for the Study of Small Groups*. Cambridge, MA: Addison-Wesley Press 1950.

195. Zimmermann C, Del Piccolo L, Bensing J, et al. Coding patient emotional cues and concerns in medical consultations: The Verona coding definitions of emotional sequences (VR-CoDES). *Patient Educ Couns* 2011;82(2):141–8. https://doi.org/S0738-3991(10)00168-0 [pii]10.1016/j.pec.2010.03.017.

196. Del Piccolo L, de Haes H, Heaven C, et al. Development of the Verona coding definitions of emotional sequences to code health providers' responses (VR-CoDES-P) to patient cues and concerns. *Patient Educ Couns* 2011;82(2):149–55. https://doi.org/S0738-3991(10)00112-6 [pii] 10.1016/j.pec.2010.02.024.

197. Roter D, Larson S. The Roter interaction analysis system (RIAS): Utility and flexibility for analysis of medical interactions. *Patient Educ Couns* 2002;46(4):243–51. https://doi.org/10.1016/S0738-3991(02)00012-5.

198. Zandbelt LC, Smets EM, Oort FJ, et al. Coding patient-centred behaviour in the medical encounter. *Soc Sci Med* 2005;61(3):661–71. https://doi.org/10.1016/j.socscimed.2004.12.006.

199. Heaven C, Clegg J, Maguire P. Transfer of communication skills training from workshop to workpace: The impact of clinical supervision. *Patient Educ Couns* 2006;60(3):313–25. https://doi.org/10.1016/j.pec.2005.08.008.

200. Roter DL, Hall JA, Blanch-Hartigan D, et al. Slicing it thin: New methods for brief sampling analysis using RIAS-coded medical dialogue. *Patient Educ Couns* 2011;82(3):410–9. https://doi.org/10.1016/j.pec.2010.11.019.

201. Plum A. Communication as skill – A critique and alternative proposal. *J Humanistic Psychol* 1981;21(4):3–19.

202. Egener B, Cole-Kelly K. Satisfying the patient, but failing the test. *Acad Med* 2004;79(6):508–10.

203. Zoppi K, Epstein RM. Is communication a skill? Communication behaviors and being in relation. *Fam Med* 2002;34(5):319–24.

204. Skelton JR. Everything you were afraid to ask about communication skills. *Br J Gen Pract* 2005;55(510):40–6.

205. Salmon P, Young B. Core assumptions and research opportunities in clinical communication. *Patient Educ Couns* 2005;58(3):225–34.

206. Salmon P, Young B. Creativity in clinical communication: From communication skills to skilled communication. *Med Educ* 2011;45(3):217–26. https://doi.org/10.1111/j.1365-2923.2010.03801.x.

207. Quirk M, Mazor K, Haley HL, et al. How patients perceive a doctor's caring attitude. *Patient Educ Couns* 2008;72(3):359–66. https://doi.org/S0738-3991(08)00270-X [pii]10.1016/j.pec.2008.05.022.

208. Bourquin C, Stiefel F. What symptoms tell us: A multiple case study of oncology consultations. *Palliat Support Care* 2021;19(4):421–36. https://doi.org/10.1017/S1478951520000899.

209. Salvade H, Stiefel F, Bourquin C. 'You'll need to settle your affairs': How the subject of death is approached by oncologists and advanced cancer patients in follow-up consultations. *Palliat Support Care* 2022:1–9. https://doi.org/10.1017/S147895152200147X.

210. Boudreau D, Wykretowicz H, Kinsella EA, et al. Discovering clinical phronesis. *Med Health Care Philos* 2024;27(2):165–79.

211. Makoul G. The SEGUE Framework for teaching and assessing communication skills. *Patient Educ Couns* 2001;45(1):23–34.

212. Hulsman RL. Shifting goals in medical communication: Determinants of goal detection and response formation. *Patient Educ Couns* 2009;74(3):302–8. https://doi.org/S0738-3991(08)00643-5 [pii]10.1016/j.pec.2008.12.001.

213. Veldhuijzen W, Mogendorff K, Ram P, et al. How doctors move from generic goals to specific communicative behavior in real practice consultations. *Patient Educ Couns* 2013;90(2):170–6. https://doi.org/10.1016/j.pec.2012.10.005.

214. Langewitz W, Nübling M, Weber H. A theory-based approach to analysing conversation sequences. *Epidemiol Psichiatr Soc* 2003;12(2):103–8. https://doi.org/10.1017/S1121189X00006163.

215. Stiles WB. Evaluating medical interview process components: Null correlations with outcomes may be misleading. *Med Care* 1989;27(2): 212–20.

216. Moore PM, Rivera S, Bravo-Soto GA, et al. Communication skills training for healthcare professionals working with people who have cancer. *Cochrane Database Syst Rev* 2018;7:CD003751. https://doi.org/10.1002/ 14651858.CD003751.pub4.

217. Uitterhoeve RJ, Bensing JM, Grol RP, et al. The effect of communication skills training on patient outcomes in cancer care: A systematic review of the literature. *Eur J Cancer Care (Engl)* 2010;19(4):442–57. https://doi.org/ ECC1082 [pii]10.1111/j.1365–2354.2009.01082.x.

218. Barth J, Lannen P. Efficacy of communication skills training courses in oncology: A systematic review and meta-analysis. *Ann Oncol* 2011;22 (5):1030–40. https://doi.org/10.1093/annonc/mdq441.

219. Selman LE, Brighton LJ, Hawkins A, et al. The effect of communication skills training for generalist palliative care providers on patient-reported outcomes and clinician behaviors: A systematic review and meta-analysis. *J Pain Symptom Manage* 2017;54(3):404–16. https://doi.org/10.1016/ j.jpainsymman.2017.04.007.

220. Gilligan C, Powell M, Lynagh MC, et al. Interventions for improving medical students' interpersonal communication in medical consultations. *Cochrane Database Syst Rev* 2021(2):CD012418. https://doi.org/ 10.1002/14651858.CD012418.pub2.

221. Salmon P, Mendick N, Young B. Integrative qualitative communication analysis of consultation and patient and practitioner perspectives: Towards a theory of authentic caring in clinical relationships. *Patient Educ Couns* 2011;82(3):448–54. https://doi.org/S0738-3991(10)00625-7 [pii]10.1016/j.pec.2010.10.017.

222. Alexander HA. Human agency and the curriculum. *Theory Res Educ* 2005;3:343–69.

223. Hillen MA, de Haes HC, Stalpers LJ, et al. How can communication by oncologists enhance patients' trust? An experimental study. *Ann Oncol* 2014;25(4):896–901. https://doi.org/10.1093/annonc/mdu027.

224. Eisner EW. What can education learn from the arts about the practice of education? *Int J Educ Arts* 2004;5(4):1–12.

225. Fallowfield L, Jenkins V, Farewell V, et al. Efficacy of a cancer research UK communication skills training model for oncologists: A randomised controlled trial. *Lancet* 2002;359(9307):650–6. https://doi.org/S0140-6736(02)07810-8 [pii]10.1016/S0140-6736(02)07810-8.

226. Fallowfield L, Jenkins V, Farewell V, et al. Enduring impact of communication skills training: Results of a 12-month follow-up. *Br J Cancer* 2003;89(8):1445–9. https://doi.org/10.1038/sj.bjc.6601309.

227. Fallowfield L, Jenkins V. Current concepts of communication skills training in oncology. *Recent Results Cancer Res* 2006;168:105–12.

228. Hatem D, Mazor K, Fischer M, et al. Applying patient perspectives on caring to curriculum development. *Patient Educ Couns* 2008;72-(3):367–73. https://doi.org/S0738-3991(08)00268-1 [pii]10.1016/j.pec.2008.05.020.

229. Epstein RM. Making communication research matter: What do patients notice, what do patients want, and what do patients need? *Patient Educ Couns* 2006;60(3):272–8.

230. Burt J, Abel G, Elmore N, et al. Rating communication in GP consultations: The association between ratings made by patients and trained clinical raters. *Med Care Res Rev* 2018;75(2):201–18. https://doi.org/10.1177/1077558716671217.

231. Hulsman RL, Ros WJ, Winnubst JA, et al. The effectiveness of a computer-assisted instruction programme on communication skills of medical specialists in oncology. *Med Educ* 2002;36(2):125–34.

232. Agledahl KM, Gulbrandsen Pl, FÃ¸rde R, et al. Courteous but not curious: How doctors' politeness masks their existential neglect: A qualitative study of video-recorded patient consultations. *J Med Ethics* 2011;37(11):650–4. https://doi.org/10.1136/jme.2010.041988.

233. Curtis JR, Back AL, Ford DW, et al. Effect of communication skills training for residents and nurse practitioners on quality of communication with patients with serious illness: A randomized trial. *JAMA* 2013;310(21):2271–81. https://doi.org/10.1001/jama.2013.282081.

234. Essers G, van Dulmen S, van Weel C, et al. Identifying context factors explaining physician's low performance in communication assessment: An explorative study in general practice. *BMC Fam Pract* 2011;12:1–8. https://doi.org/13810.1186/1471-2296-12-138.

235. Cocksedge S, May C. The listening loop: A model of choice about cues within primary care consultations. *Med Educ* 2005;39(10):999–1005.

236. Robinson WD, Priest LA, Susman JL, et al. Technician, friend, detective, and healer: family physicians' responses to emotional distress. *J Fam Pract* 2001;50(10):864–70.

237. Salander P, Sandström M. A Balint-inspired reflective forum in oncology for medical residents: Main themes during seven years. *Patient Educ Couns* 2014;97(1):47–51. http://dx.doi.org/10.1016/j.pec.2014.06.008.

238. Stiefel F, Nakamura K, Ishitani K, et al. Collusion in palliative care: An exploratory study with the Collusion Classification Grid. *Palliat Support Care* 2019;17(6):637–42. https://doi.org/10.1017/S1478951519000142.

239. Grignoli N, Wullschleger R, Di Bernardo V, et al. Hope and therapeutic privilege: Time for shared prognosis communication. *J Med Ethics* 2021;47(12):e47. https://doi.org/10.1136/medethics-2020-106157.

240. Stiefel F, Nakamura K, Terui T, et al. Collusions between patients and clinicians in end-of-life care: Why clarity matters. *J Pain Symptom Manage* 2017;53(4):776–82. https://doi.org/10.1016/j.jpainsymman.2016.11.011.

241. Baile WF, Buckman R, Lenzi R, et al. SPIKES-A six-step protocol for delivering bad news: Application to the patient with cancer. *Oncologist* 2000;5(4):302–11. https://doi.org/10.1634/theoncologist.5-4-302.

242. Langewitz W. Breaking bad news-Quo vadis? *Patient Educ Couns* 2017;100(4):607–09. https://doi.org/10.1016/j.pec.2017.03.002.

243. Eggly S, Penner L, Albrecht TL, et al. Discussing bad news in the outpatient oncology clinic: Rethinking current communication guidelines. *J Clin Oncol* 2006;24(4):716–9. https://doi.org/10.1200/jco.2005.03.0577.

244. Salander P. Bad news from the patient's perspective: An analysis of the written narratives of newly diagnosed cancer patients. *Soc Sci Med* 2002;55(5):721–32.

245. Salander P. Patients with cancer react differently – Training in breaking bad news can therefore not be reduced to learning pre-defined behaviours. *Patient Educ Couns* 2017;100(10):1955–6. https://doi.org/10.1016/j.pec.2017.05.025.

246. Nettleton S. 'I just want permission to be ill': Towards a sociology of medically unexplained symptoms. *Soc Sci Med* 2006;62(5):1167–78.

247. Mendick N, Young B, Holcombe C, et al. The 'information spectrum': A qualitative study of how breast cancer surgeons give information and of how their patients experience it. *Psychooncology* 2013;22(10):2364–71. https://doi.org/10.1002/pon.3301.

248. Mendick N, Young B, Holcombe C, et al. How do surgeons think they learn about communication? A qualitative study. *Med Educ* 2015;49 (4):408–16. https://doi.org/10.1111/medu.12648.

249. Mahendiran M, Yeung H, Rossi S. Evaluating the effectiveness of the SPIKES model to break bad news – A systematic review. *Am J Hosp Palliat Care* 2023;40:1231–60. https://doi.org/10.1177/1049909122 1146296.

250. Paul CL, Clinton-McHarg T, Sanson-Fisher RW, et al. Are we there yet? The state of the evidence base for guidelines on breaking bad news to

cancer patients. *Eur J Cancer* 2009;45(17):2960–6. https://doi.org/S0959-8049(09)00650-9 [pii]10.1016/j.ejca.2009.08.013.

251. Salmon P, Young B. How could we know if communication skills training needed no more evaluation? The case for rigour in research design. *Patient Educ Couns* 2019;102(8):1401–3. https://doi.org/10.1016/j.pec.2019.05.026.

252. Bylund CL, Banerjee SC, Bialer PA, et al. A rigorous evaluation of an institutionally-based communication skills program for post-graduate oncology trainees. *Patient Educ Couns* 2018;101(11):1924–33. https://doi.org/10.1016/j.pec.2018.05.026.

253. Girgis A, Cockburn J, Butow P, et al. Improving patient emotional functioning and psychological morbidity: Evaluation of a consultation skills training program for oncologists. *Patient Educ Couns* 2009;77(3):456–62. https://doi.org/10.1016/j.pec.2009.09.018.

254. Pehrson C, Banerjee SC, Manna R, et al. Responding empathically to patients: Development, implementation, and evaluation of a communication skills training module for oncology nurses. *Patient Educ Couns* 2016;99(4):610–6. https://doi.org/10.1016/j.pec.2015.11.021.

255. Beckman HB, Frankel RM. The effect of physician behavior on the collection of data. *Ann Intern Med* 1984;101(5):692–6. https://doi.org/10.7326/0003-4819-101-5-692.

256. Thom R, Silbersweig DA, Boland RJ. Major depressive disorder in medical illness: A review of assessment, prevalence, and treatment options. *Psychosom Med* 2019;81(3):246–55. https://doi.org/10.1097/PSY.0000000000000678.

257. Grassi L, Caruso R, Riba MB, et al. Anxiety and depression in adult cancer patients: ESMO Clinical Practice Guideline. *ESMO Open* 2023;8(2):101155. https://doi.org/10.1016/j.esmoop.2023.101155.

258. Brandenbarg D, Maass S, Geerse OP, et al. A systematic review on the prevalence of symptoms of depression, anxiety and distress in long-term cancer survivors: Implications for primary care. *Eur J Cancer Care (Engl)* 2019;28(3):e13086. https://doi.org/10.1111/ecc.13086.

259. Swartzman S, Booth JN, Munro A, et al. Posttraumatic stress disorder after cancer diagnosis in adults: A meta-analysis. *Depress Anxiety* 2017;34(4):327–39. https://doi.org/10.1002/da.22542.

260. Al Maqbali M, Al Sinani M, Al Naamani Z, et al. Prevalence of fatigue in patients with cancer: A systematic review and meta-analysis. *J Pain Symptom Manage* 2021;61(1):167–89.e14. https://doi.org/10.1016/j.jpainsymman.2020.07.037.

261. Jones JM, Olson K, Catton P, et al. Cancer-related fatigue and associated disability in post-treatment cancer survivors. *J Cancer Surviv* 2016;10 (1):51–61. https://doi.org/10.1007/s11764-015-0450-2.

262. Reuter K, Harter M. The concepts of fatigue and depression in cancer. *Eur J Cancer Care* 2004;13(2):127–34. https://doi.org/10.1111/j.1365-2354.2003.00464.x.

263. Lee C-H, Giuliani F. The role of inflammation in depression and fatigue. *Front Immunol* 2019;10:1696. https://doi.org/10.3389/fimmu.2019.01696.

264. Politynska B, Pokorska O, Wojtukiewicz AM, et al. Is depression the missing link between inflammatory mediators and cancer? *Pharmacol Ther* 2022;240:108293. https://doi.org/10.1016/j.pharmthera.2022.108293.

265. Salmon P, Hill J, Krespi R, et al. The role of child abuse and age in vulnerability to emotional problems after surgery for breast cancer. *Eur J Cancer* 2006;42(15):2517–23.

266. Locock L, Ziébland S. Mike bury: Biographical disruption and long-term and other health conditions. In Collyer F, ed. *The Palgrave Handbook of Social Theory in Health, Illness and Medicine.* London: Palgrave Macmillan UK 2015:582–98.

267. Brennan J. *Cancer in Context.* Oxford: Oxford University Press 2004.

268. DiMatteo MR, Lepper HS, Croghan TW. Depression is a risk factor for noncompliance with medical treatment: Meta-analysis of the effects of anxiety and depression on patient adherence. *Arch Intern Med* 2000;160 (14):2101–7. https://doi.org/10.1001/archinte.160.14.2101.

269. Satin JR, Linden W, Phillips MJ. Depression as a predictor of disease progression and mortality in cancer patients: A meta-analysis. *Cancer* 2009;115(22):5349–61. https://doi.org/10.1002/cncr.24561.

270. Wang X, Wang N, Zhong L, et al. Prognostic value of depression and anxiety on breast cancer recurrence and mortality: A systematic review and meta-analysis of 282,203 patients. *Mol Psychiatry* 2020;25 (12):3186–97. https://doi.org/10.1038/s41380-020-00865-6.

271. Carlson LE, Bultz BD. Benefits of psychosocial oncology care: Improved quality of life and medical cost offset. *Health Qual Life Outcomes* 2003;1:8.

272. Gaulin M, Simard M, Candas B, et al. Combined impacts of multimorbidity and mental disorders on frequent emergency department visits: A retrospective cohort study in Quebec, Canada. *Can Med Assoc J* 2019;191(26):E724–E32. https://doi.org/10.1503/cmaj.181712.

273. Epstein RM, Street RLJ. *Patient-Centered Communication in Cancer Care: Promoting Healing and Reducing Suffering.* Bethesda, MD: National Cancer Institute, NIH 2007.

274. National Institute for Clinical Excellence. *Improving Supportive and Palliative Care for Adults with Cancer.* London: National Institute for Clinical Excellence 2004.

275. Jefford M, Tattersall MH. Informing and involving cancer patients in their own care. *Lancet Oncol* 2002;3(10):629–37. https://doi.org/10.1016/s1470-2045(02)00877-x.

276. Bultz BD, Carlson LE. Emotional distress: The sixth vital sign in cancer care. *J Clin Oncol* 2005;23(26):6440–1. https://doi.org/10.1200/jco.2005.02.3259.

277. Ownby KK. Use of the distress thermometer in clinical practice. *J Adv Pract Oncol* 2019;10(2):175–9.

278. Smith SK, Loscalzo M, Mayer C, et al. Best practices in oncology distress management: Beyond the screen. *American Society of Clinical Oncology Educational Book* 2018(38):813–21. https://doi.org/10.1200/edbk_201307.

279. Dekker J, Graves KD, Badger TA, et al. Management of distress in patients with cancer—Are we doing the right thing? *Ann Behav Med* 2021;54(12):978–84. https://doi.org/10.1093/abm/kaaa091.

280. Salmon P, Clark L, McGrath E, et al. Screening for psychological distress in cancer: renewing the research agenda. *Psychooncology* 2015;24(3):262–8. https://doi.org/10.1002/pon.3640.

281. Beesley H, Goodfellow S, Holcombe C, et al. The intensity of breast cancer patients' relationships with their surgeons after the first meeting: Evidence that relationships are not 'built' but arise from attachment processes. *Eur J Surg Oncol* 2016;42(5):679–84. https://doi.org/10.1016/j.ejso.2016.02.001.

282. Atherton K, Young B, Kalakonda N, et al. Perspectives of patients with haematological cancer on how clinicians meet their information needs: 'Managing' information versus 'giving' it. *Psychooncology* 2018;27(7):1719–26. https://doi.org/10.1002/pon.4714.

283. Lilliehorn S, Hamberg K, Kero A, et al. 'Admission into a helping plan': A watershed between positive and negative experiences in breast cancer. *Psychooncology* 2010;19(8):806–13. https://doi.org/10.1002/pon.1619.

284. Davies S, Salmon P, Young B. When trust is threatened: Qualitative study of parents' perspectives on problematic clinical relationships in child cancer care. *Psychooncology* 2017;26(9):1301–6. https://doi.org/10.1002/pon.4454.

285. Salmon P, Holcombe C, Clark L, et al. Relationships with clinical staff after a diagnosis of breast cancer are associated with patients' experience of care and abuse in childhood. *J Psychosom Res* 2007;63(3):255–62.

286. Fagundes CP, Lindgren ME, Shapiro CL, et al. Child maltreatment and breast cancer survivors: Social support makes a difference for quality of life, fatigue and cancer stress. *Eur J Cancer* 2012;48(5):728–36. https://doi.org/10.1016/j.ejca.2011.06.022.

287. Clark L, Beesley H, Holcombe C, et al. The influence of childhood abuse and adult attachment style on clinical relationships in breast cancer care. *Gen Hosp Psychiatry* 2011;33(6):579–86. https://doi.org/S0163-8343(11)00244-1[pii]10.1016/j.genhosppsych.2011.07.007.

288. Salmon P, Hill J, Ward J, et al. Faith and protection: The construction of hope by parents of children with leukemia and their oncologists. *Oncologist* 2012;17(3):398–404. https://doi.org/theoncologist.2011-0308 [pii]10.1634/theoncologist.2011–0308.

289. Salmon P, Young B. The validity of education and guidance for clinical communication in cancer care: evidence-based practice will depend on practice-based evidence. *Patient Educ Couns* 2013;90(2):193–9. https://doi.org/S0738-3991(12)00168-1 [pii]10.1016/j.pec.2012.04.010.

290. Salmon P, Young B. Qualitative methods can test and challenge what we think we know about clinical communication – if they are not too constrained by methodological 'brands'. *Patient Educ Couns* 2018;101(9):1515–7. https://doi.org/10.1016/j.pec.2018.07.005.

291. Kendall J, Glaze K, Oakland S, et al. What do 1281 distress screeners tell us about cancer patients in a community cancer center? *Psychooncology* 2011;20(6):594–600. https://doi.org/10.1002/pon.1907.

292. Helft PR. Necessary collusion: Prognostic communication with advanced cancer patients. *J Clin Oncol* 2005;23(13):3146–50.

293. Rodenbach RA, Rodenbach KE, Tejani MA, et al. Relationships between personal attitudes about death and communication with terminally ill patients: How oncology clinicians grapple with mortality. *Patient Educ Couns* 2016;99(3):356–63.

294. The AM, Hak T, Koeter G, et al. Collusion in doctor-patient communication about imminent death: An ethnographic study. *Br Med J* 2000;321(7273):1376–81.

295. Byrne A, Ellershaw J, Holcombe C, et al. Patients' experience of cancer: Evidence of the role of 'fighting' in collusive clinical communication. *Patient Educ Couns* 2002;48(1):15–21.

296. National Comprehensive Cancer Network. *Distress during Cancer Care.* Plymouth Meeting, PA: National Comprehensive Cancer Network 2024.

297. Salander P. Does advocating screening for distress in cancer rest more on ideology than on science? *Patient Educ Couns* 2017;100(5):858–60. https://doi.org/10.1016/j.pec.2016.11.009.

298. Meggiolaro E, De Padova S, Ruffilli F, et al. From distress screening to uptake: An Italian multicenter study of cancer patients. *Cancers (Basel)* 2021;13(15):3761. https://doi.org/10.3390/cancers13153761.

299. Baker P, Beesley H, Dinwoodie R, et al. 'You're putting thoughts into my head': A qualitative study of the readiness of patients with breast, lung or prostate cancer to address emotional needs through the first 18months after diagnosis. *Psychooncology* 2013;22(6):1402–10. https://doi.org/10.1002/pon.3156.

300. Atherton K, Young B, Salmon P. Understanding the information needs of people with haematological cancers: A meta-ethnography of quantitative and qualitative research. *Eur J Cancer Care* 2017;26(6):e12647. https://doi.org/10.1111/ecc.12647.

301. Leydon GM, Boulton M, Moynihan C, et al. Cancer patients' information needs and information seeking behaviour: In depth interview study. *Br Med J* 2000;320(7239):909–13.

302. Salander P, Bergenheim T, Henriksson R. The creation of protection and hope in patients with malignant brain tumours. *Soc Sci Med* 1996;42 (7):985–96.

303. Mendick N, Young B, Holcombe C, et al. Telling 'everything' but not 'too much': the surgeon's dilemma in consultations about breast cancer. *World J Surg* 2011;35(10):2187–95. https://doi.org/10.1007/s00268-011-1195-3.

304. Nissim R, Zimmermann C, Minden M, et al. Abducted by the illness: A qualitative study of traumatic stress in individuals with acute leukemia. *Leuk Res* 2013;37(5):496–502. https://doi.org/10.1016/j.leukres.2012.12.007.

305. Salander P, Bergknut M, Henriksson R. The creation of hope in patients with lung cancer. *Acta Oncol* 2014;53(9):1205–11. https://doi.org/10.3109/0284186X.2014.921725.

306. Perakyla A. Hope work in the care of seriously Ill patients. *Qual Health Res* 1991;1(4):407–33. https://doi.org/10.1177/104973239100100402.

307. Salander P. Cancer and 'playing' with reality: Clinical guidance with the help of the intermediate area and disavowal. *Acta Oncol* 2012;51(4): 541–60. https://doi.org/10.3109/0284186X.2011.639389.

308. Salander P, Windahl G. Does 'denial' really cover our everyday experiences in clinical oncology? A critical view from a psychoanalytic perspective on the use of 'denial'. *Br J Med Psychol* 1999;72 (Pt 2):267–79. https://doi.org/10.1348/000711299159899.

309. Salander P, Lilliehorn S. To carry on as before: A meta-synthesis of qualitative studies in lung cancer. *Lung Cancer* 2016;99:88–93. https://doi.org/10.1016/j.lungcan.2016.06.014.

310. Salander P. Everyday life as a bridge over troubled water. *Psychooncology* 2016;25(3):347–8. https://doi.org/10.1002/pon.3905.

311. Baker P, Beesley H, Fletcher I, et al. 'Getting back to normal' or 'a new type of normal'? A qualitative study of patients' responses to the existential threat of cancer. *Eur J Cancer Care (Engl)* 2016;25(1):180–9. https://doi.org/10.1111/ecc.12274.

312. Blakely K, Karanicolas PJ, Wright FC, et al. Optimistic honesty: Understanding surgeon and patient perspectives on hopeful communication in pancreatic cancer care. *HPB (Oxford)* 2017;19(7):611–19. https://doi.org/10.1016/j.hpb.2017.04.001.

313. Kalanithi P. How Long Have I Got Left? *New York Times (1857–1922)* 2014;163(56393):9.

314. Wilkinson S, Kitzinger C. Thinking differently about thinking positive: A discursive approach to cancer patients' talk. *Soc Sci Med* 2000;50(6):797–811. https://doi.org/S0277953699003378 [pii].

315. Leydon GM. 'Yours is potentially serious but most of these are cured': Optimistic communication in UK outpatient oncology consultations. *Psychooncology* 2008;17(11):1081–8. https://doi.org/10.1002/pon.1392.

316. Ingelfinger FJ. Arrogance. *N Engl J Med* 1980;303(26):1507–11.

317. Krathwohl DR, Bloom BS, Masia BB. *Taxonomy of Educational Objectives: The Classification of Educational Goals*. London: Longman 1964.

318. Anderson LW, Krathwohl DR, eds. *A Taxonomy for Learning, Teaching, and Assessing: A Revision of Bloom's Taxonomy of Educational Objectives*. New York: Longman 2001.

319. Simpson EJ. *The Classification of Educational Objectives in the Psycho Motor Domain*. Rockville, ERIC 1966.

320. Labrie N, Schulz PJ. Does argumentation matter? A systematic literature review on the role of argumentation in doctor-patient communication. *Health Communication* 2014;29(10):996–1008. https://doi.org/10.1080/10410236.2013.829018

321. Leontowicz J. Lost art of argumentation. *Can Med Educ J* 2017;8(3):e121–e2.

322. Bigi S. The role of argumentative strategies in the construction of emergent common ground in a patient-centered approach to the medical encounter. *J Argum Context* 2018;7(2):141–56.

323. Wilkinson SR. *Coping and Complaining: Attachment and the Language of Disease*. Hove: Brunner-Routledge 2003.

324. Salmon P, Young B. Is clinical communication the one area of clinical oncology that needs no new ideas? *Med Educ* 2017;51(12):1291–3. https://doi.org/10.1111/medu.13373.

325. Salmon P. Conflict, collusion or collaboration in consultations about medically unexplained symptoms: The need for a curriculum of medical explanation. *Patient Educ Couns* 2007;67:246–54.

326. Plews-Ogan M, Sharpe KE. Phronesis in medical practice: The will and the skill needed to do the right thing. In Brown MEL, Veen M, Finn GM, eds. *Applied Philosophy for Health Professions Education: A Journey towards Mutual Understanding.* Singapore: Springer Nature Singapore 2022:293–309.

327. Kaldjian LC, Yoon J, Ark TK, et al. Practical wisdom in medicine through the eyes of medical students and physicians. *Med Educ* 2023;57 (12):1219–29.

328. Haidet P. Jazz and the 'art' of medicine: Improvisation in the medical encounter. *Ann Fam Med* 2007;5(2):164–69. https://doi.org/10.1370/afm.624.

329. Eisner EW. Artistry in Education. *Scand J Educ Res* 2003;47(3): 373–84.

330. Jackson N, Oliver M, Shaw M, et al., eds. *Developing Creativity in Higher Education: an Imaginative Curriculum.* Abingdon: Routledge 2006.

331. Edstrom A-M. To rest assured: A study of artistic development. *Int J Educ Arts* 2008;9(3):1–25.

332. Bleakley A, Bligh J. Students learning from patients: Let's get real in medical education. *Adv Health Sci Educ Theory Pract* 2008;13(1):89–107. https://doi.org/10.1007/s10459-006-9028-0.

333. Bell K, Boshuizen HP, Scherpbier A, et al. When only the real thing will do: Junior medical students' learning from real patients. *Med Educ* 2009;43(11):1036–43. https://doi.org/MED3508[pii]10.1111/j.1365–2923.2009.03508.x.

334. Wear D, Varley JD. Rituals of verification: The role of simulation in developing and evaluating empathic communication. *Patient Educ Couns* 2008;71(2):153–6.

335. Newble D. Techniques for measuring clinical competence: Objective structured clinical examinations. *Med Educ* 2004;38(2):199–203. https://doi.org/1755 [pii].

336. Scheffer S, Muehlinghaus I, Froehmel A, et al. Assessing students' communication skills: Validation of a global rating. *Adv Health Sci Educ Theory Pract* 2008;13(5):583–92. https://doi.org/10.1007/s10459-007-9074-2.

337. Regehr G, MacRae H, Reznick RK, et al. Comparing the psychometric properties of checklists and global rating scales for assessing performance on an OSCE-format examination. *Acad Med* 1998;73(9):993–7.

338. Huntley CD, Salmon P, Fisher PL, et al. LUCAS: A theoretically informed instrument to assess clinical communication in objective structured clinical examinations. *Med Educ* 2012;46(3):267–76. https://doi.org/10.1111/j.1365-2923.2011.04162.x.

339. Regelski TA. Conclusion: An end is a beginning. In Regelski TA, Gates JT, eds. *Music Education for Changing Times: Guiding Visions for Practice.* Dordrecht: Springer 2009:188–97.

340. de Bezenac C. No pain, no gain? Motivation and self-regulation in music learning. *Int J Educ Arts* 2009;10(16):1–33.

341. Shelton W, Campo-Engelstein L. Confronting the hidden curriculum: A four-year integrated course in ethics and professionalism grounded in virtue ethics. In Jones T, Pachucki K, eds. *The Medical/Health Humanities-Politics, Programs, and Pedagogies.* Cham: Springer 2022:177–91.

342. Noble LM, Manalastas G, Viney R, et al. Does the structure of the medical consultation align with an educational model of clinical communication? A study of physicians' consultations from a postgraduate examination. *Patient Educ Couns* 2022;105(6):1449–56.

343. Giroldi E, Veldhuijzen W, Geelen K, et al. Developing skilled doctor-patient communication in the workplace: A qualitative study of the experiences of trainees and clinical supervisors. *Adv Health Sci Educ Theory Pract* 2017;22(5):1263–78. https://doi.org/10.1007/s10459-017-9765-2.

344. Rollnick S, Kinnersley P, Butler C. Context-bound communication skills training: Development of a new method. *Med Educ* 2002;36(4):377–83. https://doi.org/10.1046/j.1365-2923.2002.01174.x.

345. Doukas DJ, Ozar DT, Darragh M, et al. Virtue and care ethics & humanism in medical education: a scoping review. *BMC Med Educ* 2022;22 (1):1–10.

346. Shaw AC, McQuade JL, Reilley MJ, et al. Integrating storytelling into a communication skills teaching program for medical oncology fellows. *J Cancer Educ* 2019;34(6):1198–203. https://doi.org/10.1007/s13187-018-1428-3.

347. Wilkes M, Milgrom E, Hoffman JR. Towards more empathic medical students: A medical student hospitalization experience. *Med Educ* 2002;36(6):528–33. https://doi.org/10.1046/j.1365-2923.2002.01230.x.

348. Larson EB, Yao X. Clinical empathy as emotional labor in the patient-physician relationship. *JAMA* 2005;293(9):1100–6.

349. Finestone HM, Conter DB. Acting in medical practice. *Lancet* 1994;344 (8925):801–2.

350. Stiefel F, Nakamura K, Terui T, et al. The collusion classification grid: A supervision and research tool. *J Pain Symptom Manage* 2018;55(2):E1–E3. https://doi.org/10.1016/j.jpainsymman.2017.10.020.

351. Stiefel F, Bourquin C, Wild B, et al. Oncology clinicians' feelings towards patients presented in supervision: A pre-post assessment using the feeling word checklist. *Psychooncology* 2024;33(3):e6318. https://doi.org/10.1002/pon.6318.

352. Delany C, Benhamu J, McDougall R, et al. Supporting cancer care clinicians to 'hold' their patients during and beyond the COVID-19 pandemic: A role for reflective ethics discussions. *Intern Med J* 2021;51(7):1143–5. https://doi.org/10.1111/imj.15375.

353. Browning DM, Meyer EC, Truog RD, et al. Difficult conversations in health care: Cultivating relational learning to address the hidden curriculum. *Acad Med* 2007;82(9):905–13. https://doi.org/10.1097/ACM.0b013e31812f77b9.

354. Meyer EC, Brodsky D, Hansen AR, et al. An interdisciplinary, family-focused approach to relational learning in neonatal intensive care. *J Perinatol* 2011;31(3):212–9. https://doi.org/10.1038/jp.2010.109.

355. Lamiani G, Meyer EC, Leone D, et al. Cross-cultural adaptation of an innovative approach to learning about difficult conversations in healthcare. *Med Teach* 2011;33(2):e57–64. https://doi.org/10.3109/0142159X.2011.534207.

356. Bell SK, Pascucci R, Fancy K, et al. The educational value of improvisational actors to teach communication and relational skills: Perspectives of interprofessional learners, faculty, and actors. *Patient Educ Couns* 2014;96(3):381–8. https://doi.org/10.1016/j.pec.2014.07.001.

357. Lyon W. Virtue and medical ethics education. *Philos Ethics Humanit Med* 2021;16(1):2.

358. van den Eertwegh V, van Dulmen S, van Dalen J, et al. Learning in context: Identifying gaps in research on the transfer of medical communication skills to the clinical workplace. *Patient Educ Couns* 2013;90 (2):184–92. https://doi.org/10.1016/j.pec.2012.06.008.

359. de Bruin B, Zaal R, Jeurissen R. Pitting virtue ethics against situationism: An empirical argument for virtue. *Ethical Theory Moral Pract* 2023;26(3): 463–79.

360. Upton CL. Virtue ethics and moral psychology: The situationism debate. *J Ethics* 2009;13(2):103–15.

361. Jackson JL, Kroenke K. The effect of unmet expectations among adults presenting with physical symptoms. *Ann Intern Med* 2001;134(9 Pt 2): 889–97. https://doi.org/200105011-00013 [pii].

362. Stead L, Bergson G, Lancaster T. Physician advice for smoking cessation. *Cochrane Database Syst Rev* 2008(2):CD000165.

363. Kotzee B, Ignatowicz A. Measuring 'virtue' in medicine. *Med Health Care Philos* 2016;19:149–61.

364. Gilligan C, Bigi S, Rehman S. What constitutes an 'evidence-base' in the healthcare communication field? *Patient Educ Couns* 2023;110:107685. https://doi.org/10.1016/j.pec.2023.107685.

365. Portmann J. Like marriage, without the romance. *J Med Ethics* 2000;26 (3):194–7.

Cambridge Elements$^{\equiv}$

Health Communication

Louise Cummings
The Hong Kong Polytechnic University

Louise Cummings is Professor in the Department of English and Communication at The Hong Kong Polytechnic University. She conducts research in health communication and clinical linguistics and is the author and editor of over 20 books in these areas. Prof. Cummings is a member of the Royal College of Speech and Language Therapists and the Health & Care Professions Council in the UK.

About the Series

This series brings together a wide range of disciplines that converge on the study of communication in health settings. Each element examines a key topic in health communication and is carefully crafted by experts in their respective disciplines. The series is relevant to students, researchers, and practitioners in humanities, medical and health professions, and social scientific disciplines.

Cambridge Elements ≡

Health Communication

Elements in the Series